NCLEX-RN®

250 New-Format Questions

Second Edition

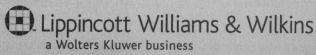

Lippincott Williams & Wilkins
a Wolters Kluwer business

Philadelphia · Baltimore · New York · London
Buenos Aires · Hong Kong · Sydney · Tokyo

STAFF

Publisher
Judith A. Schilling McCann, RN, MSN

Senior Acquisitions Editor
Elizabeth Nieginski

Editorial Director
David Moreau

Clinical Director
Joan M. Robinson, RN, MSN

Senior Art Director
Arlene Putterman

Editorial Project Manager
Jaime Stockslager Buss

Clinical Project Manager
Carol A. Saunderson. RN, BA, BS

Editors
Sid Karpoff, Jeannette Sabatini, Doris Weinstock,
Susan Williams

Clinical Editors
Tamara Kear, RN, MSN, CNN; Carol Knauff, RN, MSN, CCRN;
Anita Lockhart, RNC, MSN; Anne Marie Palatnik, MSN, APN,
BC; Barbara Stiebeling, BSN, MSN

Designers
Susan Hopkins Rodzewich (book design),
Stephanie Biddle (project manager)

Digital Composition Services
Diane Paluba (manager), Joyce Rossi Biletz,
Donna S. Morris

Manufacturing
Patricia K. Dorshaw (director), Beth J. Welsh

Editorial Assistants
Megan L. Aldinger, Karen J. Kirk, Linda K. Ruhf

Design Assistant
Georg Purvis, IV

RN2502E010106 — 021206

Library of Congress Cataloging-in-Publication Data

NCLEX-RN 250 new-format questions.—2nd ed.
   p. ; cm.
   1. Nursing—Examinations, questions, etc. 2. Nursing—Outlines, syl-
labi, etc. 3. Nurses—Licenses—United States—Examinations—Study
guides. I. Lippincott Williams & Wilkins. II. Title: NCLEX-RN two hun-
dred fifty new-format questions.
   [DNLM: 1. Nursing Care—Examination Questions. 2. Nursing—Examination Questions. WY 18.2 N339 2007]
RT55.N435 2007
610.73076—dc22
ISBN13: 978-1-58255-473-0
ISBN10: 1-58255-473-0 (alk. paper)   2005029429

Contents

Contributors | iv

How to use | v

PART **ONE**
Fundamentals of nursing | *1*

PART **TWO**
Medical-surgical nursing | *27*

PART **THREE**
Maternal-infant nursing | *75*

PART **FOUR**
Pediatric nursing | *97*

PART **FIVE**
Psychiatric and mental health nursing | *119*

Contributors

Beverly Anderson, RN, MSN
Associate Professor
Malcolm X College
Chicago, Ill.

Brandy Andrew, MSN, PNP
Assistant Nursing Professor
Northern Kentucky University
Highland Heights, Ky.

Kimberly Attwood, RN, MSN
Instructor
St. Luke's School of Nursing at Moravian College
Bethlehem, Pa.

Kathy J. Keister, RN, PhD
Assistant Professor
Miami University
Middletown, Ohio

Nancy Laplante, RN, MSN
Nursing Instructor
Neumann College
Aston, Pa.

Michelle Reeves Macaluso, RN, BSN, MN
Clinical Nurse III, Endocrinology Center
Children's Medical Center
Dallas, Tex.

Karen Madsen, RN, BSN, ADN, IBCLC
Adjunct Faculty
Labette Community College
Parsons, Kans.

Kendra S. Seiler, RN, MSN, CNOR
Nursing Instructor
Rio Hondo Community College
Whittier, Calif.

Janet Ann Smith, RN,C, MSN
Director of Nurses
Coalinga (Calif.) State Hospital

Kathleen R. Tusaie, PhD, APRN–BC
Assistant Professor of Nursing
University of Akron (Ohio)

You've worked hard to earn your degree. You're ready to move ahead in your career and begin your nursing practice. Only one thing stands in your way — the National Council Licensure Examination for Registered Nurses (NCLEX-RN).

Alternate-format questions

Every nursing student is familiar with the pressure and anxiety involved with taking the NCLEX-RN. As if the stress of the standard test questions wasn't enough, however, the National Council of State Boards of Nursing (NCSBN) added five types of alternate-format questions to the NCLEX. But don't worry, *NCLEX-RN: 250 New-Format Questions* is a cutting-edge review book that will help you become fully prepared for every type of question you may encounter on the NCLEX.

Multiple-response

The first type of alternate format is the multiple-response question. Unlike a traditional multiple-choice question, each multiple-response question can have more than one correct answer, and it may contain more than four possible answer options. You'll recognize this type of question because you'll be asked to select *all* answers that apply — not just the *best* answer (as may be requested in more traditional multiple-choice questions).

When you encounter one of these questions in this review book, read the question and all possible answers carefully. Then place check marks in the boxes next to all options that correctly answer the question. Keep in mind that you must select all correct answers for a multiple-response question to be counted as correct. On the NCLEX, there is no partial credit in the scoring of these items.

Fill-in-the-blank

The second type of alternate question format is the fill-in-the-blank question. These questions require you to provide the answer yourself, rather than select it from a list of options. For these questions, write your answer in the blank space provided after the question. Keep in mind that these questions are based on calculation problems and require only a numerical answer but no fractions. Include a decimal, if appropriate, and perform rounding at the end of the calculation, if necessary. Do not put commas within or units of measure after the numerical answer.

Hot spot

The third type of alternate format is a question in which you'll be asked to identify an area on an illustration or graphic. For these so-called "hot spot" questions, the computerized exam will ask you to place your cursor over the correct area on an illustration.

When reviewing such questions in this book, read the question and then mark an X on the illustration in the left-hand column to indicate your answer. In the right-hand column, correct answers are similarly indicated by an X on the duplicate illustration. Try to be as precise as possible when marking the location. As with the fill-in-the-blank questions, the identification questions on the computerized exam may require extremely precise answers in order for them to be considered correct.

Drag-and-drop

The fourth type of alternate format is drag-and-drop, in which you are asked to place items in a precise order. In this review book, we've supplied you with blank boxes in which you can write your answers. On the NCLEX, you will use the cursor to drag the answer options to the response boxes, where you will place them in ascending chronological order. You may also highlight each option and then click the arrow button to move the option to the answer box. Remember that *all* of your answers must appear in the correct order to be marked correct; no partial credit is given on the NCLEX.

Chart/exhibit

The fifth and final type of alternate format is called a chart/exhibit question. On the NCLEX, the computer will display two or more screens of information for you to read and will then ask a multiple-choice question related to the given materials. We have approximated this style in book form by giving you a chart or other information that you must use to answer the multiple-choice question.

About this book

The alternate-format questions are sure to make the NCLEX exam even more challenging than it has been in the past. Luckily, *NCLEX-RN: 250 New-Format Questions* was specifically developed to help you prepare for and excel at each of these types of questions. This helpful review book will boost your confidence and ease your anxiety.

A useful supplementary study guide, this book includes 250 alternate-format questions that cover all of the topics tested on the exam—including fundamentals of nursing, medical-surgical nursing, maternal-infant nursing, pediatric nursing, and psychiatric and mental health nursing. For each type of question, you'll find the correct answer as well as clear, concise rationales for correct and incorrect answers. You'll also find the associated nursing process step, client needs category and subcategory, and cognitive level.

The convenient two-column format (with questions on the left and answers on the right) enhances your preparation process by giving you instant feedback and saves you the time of flipping to the back of the book to find the correct answer.

The review questions provided in this book will test your knowledge base, improve your test-taking skills, and help you become familiar with the alternate-format question types. All of the questions in this book were written by nurses and approximate the real questions you'll find on the NCLEX.

What to expect on the NCLEX

The NCSBN has not yet established a percentage of alternate-format questions to be administered to each candidate. In fact, your exam may contain only one alternate-format question. Be confident in knowing that the questions in this book cover relevant information in a challenging manner that can be useful even if your exam doesn't include these alternate-format questions. Also, in your rush to prepare for the new-format questions, don't forget to review practice questions that follow the standard four-option, multiple-choice format. These questions will still compose the bulk of the test.

Remember that the process of testing and introducing the alternate-format questions into the NCLEX is ongoing. Because the test format is subject to change, be sure to consult the "Testing services" section of the NCSBN web site (*www.ncsbn.org*) as your exam date nears for the most up-to-date information on the NCLEX.

You've been diligently preparing for this all-important exam for years. *NCLEX-RN: 250 New-Format Questions* is the next logical step in that sound preparation, the final resource you'll need to meet the challenge of passing the NCLEX and moving on to the rewards of your nursing career. Good luck!

PART ONE

Fundamentals of nursing

Basic physical care

1. A nurse is developing a care plan for a client with an injury to the frontal lobe of the brain. Which of the following interventions should be part of the care plan?

Select all that apply.

☐ **1.** Keep instructions simple and brief because the client will have difficulty concentrating.

☐ **2.** Speak clearly and slowly because the client will have difficulty hearing.

☐ **3.** Assist with bathing because the client will have vision disturbances.

☐ **4.** Orient the client to person, place, and time as needed because of memory problems.

☐ **5.** Assess vital signs frequently because vital bodily functions are affected.

Answer: 1, 4

Rationale: Damage to the frontal lobe affects personality, memory, reasoning, concentration, and motor control of speech. Damage to the temporal lobe, not the frontal lobe, causes hearing and speech problems. Damage to the occipital lobe causes vision disturbances. Damage to the brain stem affects vital functions.

Nursing process step: Planning

Client needs category: Physiological integrity

Client needs subcategory: Basic care and comfort

Cognitive level: Application

---

2. A nurse is caring for a client with emphysema. Which of the following nursing interventions are appropriate?

Select all that apply.

☐ **1.** Reduce fluid intake to less than 2,500 ml/day.

☐ **2.** Teach diaphragmatic, pursed-lip breathing.

☐ **3.** Administer low-flow oxygen.

☐ **4.** Keep the client in a supine position as much as possible.

☐ **5.** Encourage alternating activity with rest periods.

☐ **6.** Teach use of postural drainage and chest physiotherapy.

Answer: 2, 3, 5, 6

Rationale: Diaphragmatic, pursed-lip breathing strengthens respiratory muscles and enhances oxygenation in clients with emphysema. Low-flow oxygen should be administered because a client with emphysema has chronic hypercapnia and a hypoxic respiratory drive. Alternating activity with rest allows the client to perform activities without excessive distress. If the client has difficulty mobilizing copious secretions, the nurse should teach him and his family members how to perform postural drainage and chest physiotherapy. Fluid intake should be increased to 3,000 ml/day, if not contraindicated, to liquefy secretions and facilitate their removal. The client should be placed in high-Fowler's position to improve ventilation.

Nursing process step: Planning

Client needs category: Physiological integrity

Client needs subcategory: Basic care and comfort

Cognitive level: Application

3. A nurse is caring for a client who underwent surgical repair of a detached retina in the right eye. Which of the following interventions should the nurse perform?

Select all that apply.

☐ **1.** Place the client in a prone position.

☐ **2.** Approach the client from the left side.

☐ **3.** Encourage deep breathing and coughing.

☐ **4.** Discourage bending down.

☐ **5.** Orient the client to his environment.

☐ **6.** Administer a stool softener.

Answer: 2, 4, 5, 6

Rationale: The nurse should approach the client from the left side — the unaffected side — to avoid startling him. She should also discourage the client from bending down, deep breathing, hard coughing and sneezing, and other activities that can increase intraocular pressure during the postoperative period. The client should be oriented to his environment to reduce the risk of injury. Stool softeners should be administered to discourage straining during defecation. The client should lie on his back or on the unaffected side to reduce intraocular pressure in the affected eye.

Nursing process step: Implementation

Client needs category: Physiological integrity

Client needs subcategory: Reduction of risk potential

Cognitive level: Application

---

4. A nurse is planning care for a client with hyperthyroidism. Which of the following nursing interventions are appropriate?

Select all that apply.

☐ **1.** Instill isotonic eye drops as necessary.

☐ **2.** Provide several small, well-balanced meals.

☐ **3.** Provide rest periods.

☐ **4.** Keep the environment warm.

☐ **5.** Encourage frequent visitors and conversation.

☐ **6.** Weigh the client daily.

Answer: 1, 2, 3, 6

Rationale: If the client has exophthalmos (a sign of hyperthyroidism), the conjunctivae should be moistened often with isotonic eye drops. Hyperthyroidism results in increased appetite, which can be satisfied by frequent small, well-balanced meals. The nurse should provide the client with rest periods to reduce metabolic demands. The client should be weighed daily to check for weight loss, a possible consequence of hyperthyroidism. Because metabolism is increased in hyperthyroidism, heat intolerance and excitability result. Therefore, the nurse should provide a cool and quiet environment, not a warm and busy one, to promote client comfort.

Nursing process step: Planning

Client needs category: Physiological integrity

Client needs subcategory: Basic care and comfort

Cognitive level: Application

5. A client has a tumor of the posterior pituitary gland. A nurse planning his care should include which of the following interventions?

Select all that apply.

☐ **1.** Weigh the client daily.

☐ **2.** Restrict fluids.

☐ **3.** Measure urine specific gravity.

☐ **4.** Encourage intake of coffee or tea.

☐ **5.** Monitor intake and output.

Answer: 1, 3, 5

Rationale: Tumors of the pituitary gland can lead to diabetes insipidus due to deficiency of antidiuretic hormone (ADH). Decreased ADH reduces the kidneys' ability to concentrate urine, resulting in excessive urination, thirst, and fluid intake. To monitor fluid balance, the nurse should weigh the client daily, measure urine specific gravity, and monitor intake and output. She should also encourage fluids to keep intake equal to output and prevent dehydration. Coffee, tea, and other fluids that have a diuretic effect should be avoided.

Nursing process step: Planning

Client needs category: Physiological integrity

Client needs subcategory: Basic care and comfort

Cognitive level: Application

---

6. A nurse is preparing to administer an I.M. injection in the deltoid muscle. Identify the area where the nurse would administer this injection.

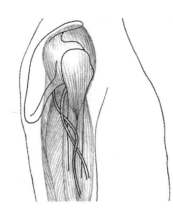

Answer:

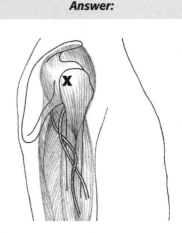

Rationale: To locate the deltoid muscle, find the lower edge of the acromial process and the point on the lateral arm in line with the axilla. The needle should be inserted 1" to 2" which is (usually two or three fingerbreadths) below the acromial process, and at a 90-degree angle, or slightly angled, toward the process.

Nursing process step: Implementation

Client needs category: Physiological integrity

Client needs subcategory: Pharmacological and parenteral therapies

Cognitive level: Application

7. A nurse is performing a fecal occult blood test using a Hemoccult slide. Place the steps for performing the fecal occult blood test in the correct order.

1. Allow the specimens to dry for 3 minutes.

2. Put on gloves.

3. Apply a drop of Hemoccult developing solution to boxes A and B on the slide's reverse side.

4. Place a stool smear on box A of the slide.

5. Apply a stool smear from another part of the specimen to box B on the slide.

6. Put a drop of Hemoccult developing solution on each control dot on the slide's reverse side.

2. Put on gloves.

4. Place a stool smear on box A of the slide.

5. Apply a stool smear from another part of the specimen to box B on the slide.

1. Allow the specimens to dry for 3 minutes.

6. Put a drop of Hemoccult developing solution on each control dot on the slide's reverse side.

3. Apply a drop of Hemoccult developing solution to boxes A and B on the slide's reverse side.

Rationale: After receiving the stool specimen from the client, the nurse should put on gloves and then follow the other steps listed above. Before using the developer, the nurse should check the expiration date; she should discard the developer if the date has expired. A blue reaction after 30 to 60 seconds indicates a positive result.

Nursing process step: Implementation

Client needs category: Health promotion and maintenance

Client needs subcategory: None

Cognitive level: Application

---

8. A nurse is caring for a client with a hiatal hernia. The client complains of abdominal pain and sternal pain after eating. The pain makes it difficult for him to sleep. Which of the following instructions should the nurse recommend when teaching this client?

Select all that apply.

☐ **1.** Avoid constrictive clothing.

☐ **2.** Lie down for 30 minutes after eating.

☐ **3.** Decrease intake of caffeine and spicy foods.

☐ **4.** Eat three meals per day.

☐ **5.** Sleep with his upper body elevated.

☐ **6.** Maintain a normal body weight.

Answer: 1, 3, 5, 6

Rationale: To reduce gastric reflux, the nurse should instruct the client to avoid constrictive clothing, caffeine, and spicy foods; sleep with his upper body elevated; lose weight, if obese; remain upright for 2 hours after eating; and eat small, frequent meals.

Nursing process step: Implementation

Client needs category: Physiological integrity

Client needs subcategory: Basic care and comfort

Cognitive level: Application

9. A nurse is assessing a client's pulses. Identify the area where the left dorsalis pedis pulse would be palpated.

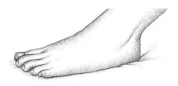

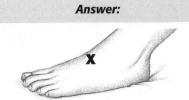

Rationale: The dorsalis pedis pulse can be palpated on the medial dorsal surface of the foot when the client's toes are pointed down. This pulse can be difficult to palpate and may seem to be absent in healthy clients.

Nursing process step: Implementation

Client needs category: Physiological integrity

Client needs subcategory: Physiological adaptation

Cognitive level: Application

---

10. A client with renal failure is placed on a potassium-restricted diet. For lunch, the client consumed 6 oz of hamburger on a bun, 1 cup of cooked broccoli, a raw pear, and iced tea. Using the chart provided, calculate how many milliequivalents of potassium were in this meal.

DIETARY SOURCES OF POTASSIUM

Foods and beverages	Serving size	Amount of potassium (mEq)
Meats		
Beef	4 oz (112 g)	11.2
Chicken	4 oz	12.0
Scallops	5 large	30.0
Vegetables		
Broccoli (cooked)	½ cup	7.0
Carrots (raw)	1 large	8.8
Potatoes (baked)	1 small	15.4
Tomatoes (raw)	1 medium	10.4
Fruits		
Bananas	1 medium	12.8
Cantaloupe	6 oz	13.0
Pears (raw)	1 medium	6.2
Beverages		
Orange juice	1 cup	11.4
Prune juice	1 cup	14.4
Tomato juice	1 cup	11.6
Milk (whole or skim)	1 cup	8.8

☐ **1.** 24.4

☐ **2.** 30

☐ **3.** 31.4

☐ **4.** 37

Answer: 4

Rationale: According to the chart, 4 oz of beef contain 11.2 mEq of potassium. Add 5.6 mEq for the additional 2 oz for a total of 16.8 mEq of potassium in the beef. The amount of potassium in 1 cup of broccoli is 14 mEq. A pear has 6.2 mEq. Thus, the total amount of potassium in this meal is 37 mEq. The iced tea and bun don't contain significant amounts of potassium and, therefore, aren't listed on the chart.

Nursing process step: Evaluation

Client needs category: Physiological integrity

Client needs subcategory: Physiological adaptation

Cognitive level: Analysis

11. A nurse is teaching a client with left leg weakness to walk with a cane. The nurse should include which of the following points about safe cane use in her client teaching?

Select all that apply.

☐ **1.** Place the cane 8″ to 10″ from the base of the little toe.

☐ **2.** Hold the cane on the uninvolved side.

☐ **3.** Adjust the cane so that the handle is level with the hip bone.

☐ **4.** Walk by moving the involved leg, then the cane, and then the uninvolved leg.

☐ **5.** Shorten the stride length on the involved side.

☐ **6.** Avoid leaning on the cane to get in and out of a chair.

Answer: 2, 3, 6

Rationale: To ambulate safely, a client with leg weakness should hold the cane in the hand opposite the involved leg with the handle level with the hip bone. The client shouldn't lean on the cane to get in or out of a chair because of the risk of falls. The cane base should be placed 4″ to 6″ from the base of the little toe. When walking, client should move the cane and involved leg simultaneously, alternating with the uninvolved leg in equal length strides and timing.

Nursing process step: Implementation

Client needs category: Physiological integrity

Client needs subcategory: Reduction of risk potential

Cognitive level: Application

---

12. A nurse is caring for a client who is recovering from an illness requiring prolonged bed rest. Based on the nursing documentation below, which of the procedures would the nurse implement next?

12/18/05	Pt. instructed in contraction of back
1015	extensors, hip extensors, knee extensors,
	and ankle flexors and extensors. Pt. able to
	demonstrate correct technique without joint
	motion or muscle lengthening. c/o being "a
	little tired" after holding each contraction
	5 seconds and repeating three times.
	Instructed to repeat exercises three times
	daily; pt. verbalized understanding of all
	information given. ———F. Brown, RN

☐ **1.** Performing active range-of-motion exercises of the legs

☐ **2.** Performing isometric exercises of the legs

☐ **3.** Providing assistance walking the client to the bathroom

☐ **4.** Performing passive range-of-motion exercises of the legs

Answer: 1

Rationale: Active range-of-motion exercises involve moving the client's joints through their full range of motion; they require some muscle strength and endurance. The client should have received passive range-of-motion exercises since admission to maintain joint flexibility and should have been taught isometric exercises to build strength and endurance for transfers and ambulation. Walking to the bathroom would be unsafe without the ability to first dangle the legs over the bedside and transfer from bed to chair.

Nursing process step: Planning

Client needs category: Physiological integrity

Client needs subcategory: Reduction of risk potential

Cognitive level: Application

Basic psychosocial needs

1. A nurse is caring for a client who is disoriented to time, place, and person and is attempting to get out of bed and pull out an I.V. line that's supplying hydration and antibiotics. The client has a vest restraint and bilateral soft wrist restraints. Which of the following actions by the nurse would be appropriate?

Select all that apply.

☐ **1.** Assess and document the behavior that requires continued use of restraints.

☐ **2.** Tie the restraints in quick-release knots.

☐ **3.** Tie the restraints to the side rails of the bed.

☐ **4.** Ask the client if he needs to go to the bathroom, and provide range-of-motion exercises every 2 hours.

☐ **5.** Position the vest restraints so that the straps are crossed in the back.

Answer: 1, 2, 4

Rationale: The client must be reassessed frequently to determine whether he is ready to have the restraints removed. This information also should be documented. Restraints should be tied in knots that can be released quickly and easily. Toileting and range-of-motion exercises should be performed every 2 hours while a client is in restraints. Restraints should never be secured to side rails because doing so can cause injury if the side rail is lowered without untying the restraint. A vest restraint should be positioned so that the straps cross in front of the client, not in the back.

Nursing process step: Implementation

Client needs category: Safe, effective care environment

Client needs subcategory: Safety and infection control

Cognitive level: Application

---

2. A client has just been diagnosed with terminal cancer and is being transferred to home hospice care. The client's daughter tells the nurse, "I don't know what to say to my mother if she asks me if she's going to die." Which of the following responses by the nurse would be appropriate?

Select all that apply.

☐ **1.** "Tell your mother not to worry. She still has some time left."

☐ **2.** "Let's talk about your mother's illness and how it will progress."

☐ **3.** "You sound like you have some questions about your mother dying. Let's talk about that."

☐ **4.** "Don't worry, hospice will take care of your mother."

☐ **5.** "Tell me how you're feeling about your mother dying."

Answer: 2, 3, 5

Rationale: Conveying information clearly and openly can alleviate fears and strengthen the individual's sense of control. Encouraging verbalization of feelings helps build a therapeutic relationship based on trust and reduces anxiety. Advising the daughter not to worry, or having her tell her mother that, ignores her feelings and discourages further communication.

Nursing process step: Implementation

Client needs category: Psychosocial integrity

Client needs subcategory: None

Cognitive level: Analysis

3. While providing care to a 26-year-old married client, a nurse notes multiple blue, purple, and yellow ecchymotic areas on her arms and trunk. When the nurse asks how she got these bruises, the client responds, "I tripped." How should the nurse respond?

Select all that apply.

☐ **1.** Document the client's statement and complete a body map indicating the size, color, shape, location, and type of injuries.

☐ **2.** Contact the local authorities to report suspicions of abuse.

☐ **3.** Assist the client in developing a safety plan for times of increased violence.

☐ **4.** Call the client's husband to arrange a meeting to discuss the situation.

☐ **5.** Tell the client that she needs to leave the abusive situation as soon as possible.

☐ **6.** Provide the client with telephone numbers of local shelters and safe houses.

Rationale: The nurse should objectively document her assessment findings. A detailed description of physical findings of abuse in the medical record is essential if legal action is pursued. All women suspected of being abuse victims should be counseled on a safety plan, which consists of recognizing escalating violence within the family, formulating a plan to exit quickly, and knowing the telephone numbers of local shelters and safe houses. The nurse should not report this suspicion of abuse because the client is a competent adult who has the right to self-determination. Contacting the client's husband without her consent violates confidentiality. The nurse should respond to the client in a nonthreatening manner that promotes trust, rather than ordering her to break off her relationship.

Nursing process step: Implementation

Client needs category: Psychosocial integrity

Client needs subcategory: None

Cognitive level: Analysis

---

4. A nurse is caring for a terminally ill client. Place the following five stages of death and dying described by Elisabeth Kübler-Ross in the order in which they occur.

| **1.** Bargaining |
| **2.** Denial and isolation |
| **3.** Acceptance |
| **4.** Anger |
| **5.** Depression |

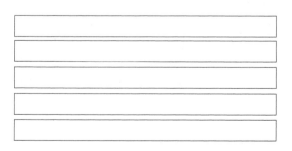

Answer:

| **2.** Denial and isolation |
| **4.** Anger |
| **1.** Bargaining |
| **5.** Depression |
| **3.** Acceptance |

Rationale: According to Kübler-Ross, the five stages of death and dying are denial and isolation, anger, bargaining, depression, and acceptance.

Nursing process step: Assessment

Client needs category: Psychosocial integrity

Client needs subcategory: None

Cognitive level: Analysis

5. A 26-year-old client with chronic renal failure was recently told by his physician that he is a poor candidate for a transplant because of chronic uncontrolled hypertension and diabetes mellitus. Now the client tells the nurse, "I want to go off dialysis. I'd rather not live than be on this treatment for the rest of my life." Which of the following responses is appropriate?

Select all that apply.

☐ **1.** Take a seat next to the client and sit quietly to reflect on what he said.

☐ **2.** Say to the client, "We all have days when we don't feel like going on."

☐ **3.** Leave the room to allow the client privacy to collect his thoughts.

☐ **4.** Say to the client, "You're feeling upset about the news you got about the transplant."

☐ **5.** Say to the client, "The treatments are only 3 days a week. You can live with that."

Answer: 1, 4

Rationale: Silence is a therapeutic communication technique that allows the nurse and client to reflect on what has taken place or been said. By waiting quietly and attentively, the nurse encourages the client to initiate and maintain a conversation. By reflecting the client's implied feelings, the nurse promotes communication. Using such platitudes as "We all have days when we don't feel like going on" fails to address the client's needs. The nurse should not leave the client alone because he may harm himself. Reminding the client of the treatment frequency doesn't address his feelings.

Nursing process step: Implementation

Client needs category: Psychosocial integrity

Client needs subcategory: None

Cognitive level: Analysis

---

6. A nurse is caring for a client with advanced cancer. After reading the nursing note below, determine the nurse's next intervention.

1/7/06	Pt. states, "The doctor says my chemotherapy
1545	isn't working anymore. They can only treat
	my symptoms now. I don't want to die in
	the hospital, I want to be in my own bed."—
	————————R. Daly, RN

☐ **1.** Reread the Patient's Bill of Rights to the client.

☐ **2.** Call the client's spouse to discuss the client's statements.

☐ **3.** Tell the client that only in the hospital can he receive adequate pain relief.

☐ **4.** Explain the use of an advance directive to express the client's wishes.

Answer: 4

Rationale: An advance directive is a legal document that's used as a guideline for life-sustaining medical care of a client with an advanced disease or disability who can no longer indicate his own wishes. This document can include a living will, which instructs the health care provider to administer no life-sustaining treatment, and a durable power of attorney for health care, which names another person to act on the client's behalf for medical decisions in the event that the client can't act for himself. The Patient's Bill of Rights is an important document but doesn't specifically address the client's wishes regarding future care. Calling the spouse is a breach of the client's right to confidentiality. Stating that only a hospital can provide adequate pain relief in a terminal situation demonstrates inadequate knowledge on the nurse's part of the resources available in the community through hospice and home care agencies in collaboration with the client's health care provider.

Nursing process step: Planning

Client needs category: Psychosocial integrity

Client needs subcategory: None

Cognitive level: Application

7. A nurse is caring for a client whose cultural background is different from her own. Which of the following actions are appropriate for the nurse to take?

Select all that apply.

- ☐ **1.** Consider that nonverbal cues, such as eye contact, may have a different meaning in different cultures.
- ☐ **2.** Respect the client's cultural beliefs.
- ☐ **3.** Ask the client if he has cultural or religious requirements that should be considered in his care.
- ☐ **4.** Explain the nurse's beliefs so that the client will understand the differences.
- ☐ **5.** Understand that all cultures experience pain in the same way.

Answer: 1, 2, 3

Rationale: Nonverbal cues may have different meanings in different cultures. In one culture, eye contact is a sign of disrespect; in another, eye contact shows respect and attentiveness. The nurse should always respect the client's cultural beliefs and ask if he has cultural or religious requirements. This may include food choices or restrictions, body coverings, or time for prayer. The nurse should attempt to understand the client's culture; it is not the client's responsibility to understand the nurse's culture. The nurse should never impose her own beliefs on her clients. Culture influences a client's experience of pain. For example, pain may be openly expressed in one culture and quietly endured in another.

Nursing process step: Planning

Client needs category: Psychosocial integrity

Client needs subcategory: None

Cognitive level: Analysis

---

8. A nurse is caring for a 45-year-old married woman who has undergone hemicolectomy for colon cancer. The woman has two children. Which of the following concepts about families should the nurse keep in mind when providing care for this client?

Select all that apply.

- ☐ **1.** Illness in one family member can affect all members.
- ☐ **2.** Family roles don't change because of illness.
- ☐ **3.** A family member may perform more than one role at a time.
- ☐ **4.** Children typically aren't affected by adult illness.
- ☐ **5.** The effects of an illness on a family depend on the stage of the family's life cycle.
- ☐ **6.** Changes in sleeping and eating patterns may be signs of stress in a family.

Answer: 1, 3, 5, 6

Rationale: Illness in one family member can affect all family members, even children. Each member of a family may have several roles to perform. A middle-aged woman, for example, may have the roles of mother, wife, wage-earner, and housekeeper. When one family member can't fulfill a role because of illness, the roles of the other family members are affected. Families move through certain predictable life cycles (such as birth of a baby, a growing family, adult children leaving home, and grandparenting). The impact of illness on the family depends on the stage of the life cycle as family members take on different roles and the family structure changes. Illness produces stress in families; changes in eating and sleeping patterns are signs of stress.

Nursing process step: Implementation

Client needs category: Health promotion and maintenance

Client needs subcategory: None

Cognitive level: Analysis

9. A nurse is assessing a newly admitted client. In the family assessment, whom should the nurse consider to be a part of the client's family?

Select all that apply.

☐ **1.** People related by blood or marriage

☐ **2.** People whom the client views as family

☐ **3.** People who live in the same house

☐ **4.** People whom the nurse thinks are important to the client

☐ **5.** People of the same racial background who live in the same house as the client

☐ **6.** People who provide for the physical and emotional needs of the client

Answer: 2, 6

Rationale: When providing care to a client, the nurse should consider family members to be all the people whom the client views as family. Family members may also include those people who provide for the physical and emotional needs of the client. The traditional definition of a family has changed and may include people not related by blood or marriage, those of a different racial background, and those who may not live in the same house as the client. Family members are defined by the client, not by the nurse.

Nursing process step: Assessment

Client needs category: Health promotion and maintenance

Client needs subcategory: None

Cognitive level: Analysis

---

10. A nurse is working with the family of a client who has Alzheimer's disease. The nurse notes that the client's spouse is too exhausted to continue providing care all alone. The adult children live too far away to provide relief on a weekly basis. Which nursing interventions would be most helpful?

Select all that apply.

☐ **1.** Calling a family meeting to tell the absent children that they must participate in caregiving

☐ **2.** Suggesting that the spouse seek psychological counseling to help cope with exhaustion

☐ **3.** Recommending community resources for adult day care and respite care

☐ **4.** Encouraging the spouse to talk about the difficulties involved in caring for a loved one

☐ **5.** Asking whether friends or church members can help with errands or provide short periods of relief

☐ **6.** Recommending that the client be placed in a long-term care facility

Answer: 3, 4, 5

Rationale: Many community services exist for Alzheimer's clients and their families. Encouraging use of these resources may make it possible to keep the client at home and to alleviate the spouse's exhaustion. The nurse can also support the caregiver by urging her to talk about the difficulties she's facing in caring for her spouse. Friends and church members may be able to help provide care to the client, allowing the caregiver time for rest, exercise, or an enjoyable activity. Arranging a family meeting to tell the children to participate more would probably be ineffective and might evoke anger or guilt. Counseling might be helpful, but it wouldn't alleviate the caregiver's physical exhaustion or address the client's immediate needs. A long-term care facility is not an option until the family is ready to make that decision.

Nursing process step: Implementation

Client needs category: Psychosocial integrity

Client needs subcategory: None

Cognitive level: Analysis

Medication and I.V. administration

1. A physician prescribes I.V. normal saline solution to be infused at a rate of 150 ml/hour for a client admitted with dehydration and pneumonia. How many liters of solution will the client receive during an 8-hour shift?

_____

Rationale: The ordered infusion rate is 150 ml/hour. The nurse should multiply 150 ml by 8 hours to determine the total volume in milliliters the client will receive during an 8-hour shift (1,200 ml). Then she should convert milliliters to liters by dividing by 1,000. The total volume in liters that the client will receive in 8 hours is 1.2 L.

Nursing process step: Planning

Client needs category: Physiological integrity

Client needs subcategory: Pharmacological and parenteral therapies

Cognitive level: Analysis

---

2. A client is prescribed heparin 6,000 units subcutaneously every 12 hours for deep vein thrombosis prophylaxis. The pharmacy dispenses a vial containing 10,000 units/1 ml. How many milliliters of heparin should the nurse administer?

_____

Rationale: The dose dispensed by the pharmacy is 10,000 units/1 ml and the desired dose is 6,000 units. The nurse should must the following equations to determine the amount of heparin to administer:

Dose on hand/Quantity on hand = Dose desired/X

10,000 units/1 ml = 6,000 units/X

10,000 units (X) = 6,000 units (ml)

X = 6,000 units (ml)/10,000 units

X = 0.6 ml.

Nursing process step: Planning

Client needs category: Physiological integrity

Client needs subcategory: Pharmacological and parenteral therapies

Cognitive level: Analysis

3. A nurse is ordered to administer ampicillin (Polycillin) 125 mg I.M. every 6 hours to a 10-kg child with a respiratory tract infection. The drug label reads, "The recommended dose for a client weighing less than 40 kg is 25 to 50 mg/kg/day I.M. or I.V. in equally divided doses at 6- to 8-hour intervals." The drug concentration is 125 mg/5 ml. Which nursing interventions are appropriate at this time?

Select all that apply.

☐ **1.** Draw up 10 ml of ampicillin to administer.

☐ **2.** Administer the medication at 10 a.m., 2 p.m., 6 p.m., and 10 p.m.

☐ **3.** Assess the client for allergies to penicillin.

☐ **4.** Administer the medication because the dosage is within the recommended range.

☐ **5.** Question the prescriber about the order because it's for more than the recommended dosage.

☐ **6.** Obtain a sputum culture, if ordered, before administering the medication.

Rationale: Because ampicillin is a penicillin antibiotic, the nurse should assess the client for penicillin allergies before administering this drug. The ampicillin dose is within the recommended range for a 10-kg client: 50 mg/kg × 10 kg = 500 mg. A dose of 500 mg divided by four (given every 6 hours) = 125 mg. Cultures should be obtained before antibiotics are given. The nurse should draw up 5 ml — not 10 ml — to administer the correct dose, according to the concentration on the label. The correct dosing schedule is every 6 to 8 hours, not every 4 hours.

Nursing process step: Implementation

Client needs category: Physiological integrity

Client needs subcategory: Pharmacological and parenteral therapies

Cognitive level: Analysis

---

4. A cardiologist prescribes digoxin (Lanoxin) 125 mcg by mouth every morning for a client diagnosed with heart failure. The pharmacy dispenses tablets that contain 0.25 mg each. How many tablets should the nurse administer in each dose?

_____

Rationale: The nurse should begin by converting 125 mcg to milligrams:

$$125 \text{ mcg}/1,000 = 0.125 \text{ mg.}$$

Then she should use the following formula to calculate the drug dosage:

Dose on hand/Quantity on hand = Dose desired/X

$$0.25 \text{ mg}/1 = 0.125 \text{ mg}/1 \text{ tablet}$$

$$0.25X = 0.125$$

$$X = 0.5 \text{ tablet.}$$

Nursing process step: Implementation

Client needs category: Physiological integrity

Client needs subcategory: Pharmacological and parenteral therapies

Cognitive level: Analysis

5. A 75-year-old client is admitted to the hospital with lower GI bleeding. His hemoglobin on admission to the emergency department is 7.3 g/dl. The physician prescribes 2 units of packed red blood cells to infuse over 2 hours each. The blood administration set has a drip factor of 10 gtt/ml. What is the flow rate in drops per minute?

_____

Answer: 21

Rationale: Each unit of packed red blood cells contains 250 ml, which should infuse over 2 hours (120 minutes). Therefore, the rate per minute is:

$$250 \text{ ml}/120 \text{ minutes} = 2.08 \text{ ml/minute}.$$

Multiply this rate by the drip factor to determine the flow rate:

$$2.08 \text{ ml} \times 10 \text{ gtt} = 20.8 \text{ gtt/minute (round up to } 21 \text{ gtt/minute)}.$$

Nursing process step: Implementation

Client needs category: Physiological integrity

Client needs subcategory: Pharmacological and parenteral therapies

Cognitive level: Analysis

---

6. A nurse is preparing a teaching plan for a client who was prescribed enalapril maleate (Vasotec) for treatment of hypertension. Which of the following instructions should the nurse include in the teaching plan?

Select all that apply.

☐ **1.** Instruct the client to avoid salt substitutes.

☐ **2.** Tell the client that light-headedness is a common adverse effect that need not be reported.

☐ **3.** Inform the client that he may have a sore throat for the first few days of therapy.

☐ **4.** Advise the client to report facial swelling or difficulty breathing immediately.

☐ **5.** Tell the client that blood tests will be necessary every 3 weeks for 2 months and periodically after that.

☐ **6.** Advise the client not to change position suddenly to minimize orthostatic hypotension.

Answer: 1, 4, 6

Rationale: When teaching the client about enalapril maleate, the nurse should tell him to avoid salt substitutes because they may contain potassium, which can cause light-headedness and syncope. Facial swelling or difficulty breathing should be reported immediately because they may be signs of angioedema, which would require discontinuation of the drug. The client should also be advised to change position slowly to minimize orthostatic hypotension. The nurse should tell the client to report light-headedness, especially in the first few days of therapy, so dosage adjustments can be made. The client should also report signs of infection, such as sore throat and fever, because the drug may decrease the white blood cell (WBC) count. Because this effect is generally seen within 3 months, the WBC count and differential should be monitored periodically.

Nursing process step: Planning

Client needs category: Physiological integrity

Client needs subcategory: Pharmacological and parenteral therapies

Cognitive level: Application

7. After sustaining a closed head injury, a client is prescribed phenytoin (Dilantin) 100 mg I.V. every 8 hours for seizure prophylaxis. Which nursing interventions are necessary when administering phenytoin?

Select all that apply.

☐ **1.** Administer phenytoin through any peripheral I.V. site.

☐ **2.** Mix I.V. doses in mixtures containing dextrose 5% in water.

☐ **3.** Administer an I.V. bolus no faster than 50 mg/minute.

☐ **4.** Monitor electrocardiogram (ECG), blood pressure, and respiratory status continuously when administering phenytoin I.V.

☐ **5.** Don't use an inline filter when administering the drug.

☐ **6.** Know that early toxicity may cause drowsiness, nausea, vomiting, nystagmus, ataxia, dysarthria, tremor, and slurred speech.

Answer: 3, 4, 6

Rationale: Administer an I.V. bolus by slow (50 mg/minute) I.V. push; too rapid an injection may cause hypotension and circulatory collapse. Continuous monitoring of ECG, blood pressure, and respiratory status is essential when administering phenytoin I.V. Early toxicity may cause drowsiness, nausea, vomiting, nystagmus, ataxia, dysarthria, tremor, and slurred speech. Later effects may include hypotension, arrhythmias, respiratory depression, and coma. Death is caused by respiratory and circulatory depression. Phenytoin shouldn't be administered by I.V. push in veins on the back of the hand; larger veins are needed to prevent discoloration associated with purple glove syndrome. Mix I.V. doses in normal saline solution and use within 30 minutes; doses mixed in dextrose 5% in water will precipitate. Use of an inline filter is recommended.

Nursing process step: Implementation

Client needs category: Physiological integrity

Client needs subcategory: Pharmacological and parenteral therapies

Cognitive level: Application

---

8. A 53-year-old client returns to his room from the postanesthesia care unit after undergoing right hemicolectomy. The physician orders 1 L of dextrose 5% in half-normal saline solution to infuse I.V. at 125 ml/hour. The drip factor of the available I.V. tubing is 15 gtt/ml. What is the drip rate in drops per minute?

Answer: 31

Rationale: The flow rate is 125 ml/hour or 125 ml/60 minutes. Use the following equation to determine the drip rate:

$$125 \text{ ml}/60 \text{ minutes} \times 15 \text{ gtt}/1 \text{ ml} =$$
$$31.25 \text{ gtt/minute (round down to 31 gtt/minute)}.$$

Nursing process step: Implementation

Client needs category: Physiological integrity

Client needs subcategory: Pharmacological and parenteral therapies

Cognitive level: Application

---

9. A physician prescribes heparin 25,000 units in 250 ml of normal saline solution to infuse I.V. at 600 units/hour for a client who suffered an acute myocardial infarction. After 6 hours of heparin therapy, the client's partial thromboplastin time is subtherapeutic. The physician orders an increase in the infusion to 800 units/hour. The nurse should set the infusion pump to deliver how many milliliters per hour?

_____

Answer: 8

Rationale: The nurse should calculate the infusion rate using the following formula:

Dose on hand/Quantity on hand = Dose desired/X

25,000 units/250 ml = 800 units/hour/X

25,000 units (X) = 250 ml (800 units/hour)

25,000 X = 200,000 ml/hour

X = 8 ml/hour.

Nursing process step: Implementation

Client needs category: Physiological integrity

Client needs subcategory: Pharmacological and parenteral therapies

Cognitive level: Application

---

10. After undergoing small-bowel resection, a client is prescribed metronidazole (Flagyl) 500 mg I.V. The mixed I.V. solution contains 100 ml. The nurse is to administer the drug over 30 minutes. The drip factor of the available I.V. tubing is 15 gtt/ml. What is the drip rate in drops per minute?

_____

Answer: 50

Rationale: The nurse should use the following equation to calculate the drip rate:

Total quantity/Administration time × gtt/min = X

100 ml/30 min × 15 gtt/min = X

$$X = \frac{1500 \text{ gtt}}{30 \text{ minute}}$$

X = 50 gtt/minute.

Nursing process step: Implementation

Client needs category: Physiological integrity

Client needs subcategory: Pharmacological and parenteral therapies

Cognitive level: Application

11. A client with an I.V. line in place complains of pain at the insertion site. Assessment of the site reveals a vein that's red, warm, and hard. Which of the following actions should the nurse take?

Select all that apply.

☐ **1.** Slow the infusion rate while notifying the prescriber.

☐ **2.** Discontinue the infusion at the affected site.

☐ **3.** Restart the infusion distal to the discontinued I.V. site.

☐ **4.** Assess the client for skin sloughing.

☐ **5.** Apply warm soaks to the I.V. site.

☐ **6.** Document the assessment, nurses' actions, and client's responses.

Answer: 2, 5, 6

Rationale: Redness, warmth, pain, and a hard, cord-like vein at the I.V. insertion site suggest that the client has phlebitis. The nurse should discontinue the I.V. infusion and insert a new I.V. catheter proximal to or above the discontinued site or in the other arm. Applying warm soaks to the site reduces inflammation. The nurse should document the assessment of the I.V. site, actions taken, and client's response to the situation. Slowing the infusion rate won't reduce the phlebitis. Restarting the infusion at a site distal to the phlebitis may contribute to the inflammation. Skin sloughing isn't a symptom of phlebitis; it's associated with extravasation of certain toxic medications.

Nursing process step: Implementation

Client needs category: Physiological integrity

Client needs subcategory: Pharmacological and parenteral therapies

Cognitive level: Application

---

12. After suffering an acute myocardial infarction (MI), a client with a history of type 1 diabetes is prescribed metoprolol (Lopressor) I.V. Which nursing interventions are associated with I.V. administration of metoprolol?

Select all that apply.

☐ **1.** Monitor glucose levels closely.

☐ **2.** Monitor for heart block and bradycardia.

☐ **3.** Monitor blood pressure closely.

☐ **4.** Mix the drug in 50 ml of dextrose 5% in water and infuse over 30 minutes.

☐ **5.** Know that the drug isn't compatible with morphine.

Answer: 1, 2, 3

Rationale: Metoprolol masks the common signs of hypoglycemia; therefore, glucose levels should be monitored closely in diabetic clients. Monitor the client for heart block or bradycardia. When used to treat an MI, metoprolol is contraindicated in clients with heart rates less than 45 beats/minute and any degree of heart block, so the nurse should monitor the client for bradycardia and heart block. Metoprolol masks common signs and symptoms of shock, such as decreased blood pressure, so blood pressure should be monitored closely. Give the drug undiluted by direct injection. Although metoprolol shouldn't be mixed with other drugs, studies have shown that it's compatible when mixed with morphine sulfate or when administered with alteplase infusion at a Y-site connection.

Nursing process step: Implementation

Client needs category: Physiological integrity

Client needs subcategory: Pharmacological and parenteral therapies

Cognitive level: Application

Basic physical assessment

1. A client who was involved in a motor vehicle accident is admitted to the intensive care unit. The emergency department admission record indicates that the client was hit in the right temporal lobe. A nurse would expect the client to demonstrate abnormalities in which of the following areas?

Select all that apply.

☐ **1.** Difficulty comprehending language

☐ **2.** Decreased hearing

☐ **3.** Aphasia

☐ **4.** Amnesia for recent events

☐ **5.** Ataxic gait

☐ **6.** Personality changes

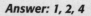
Answer: 1, 2, 4

Rationale: The temporal lobe controls hearing, language comprehension, and the storage and recall of memories. Aphasia and personality changes might be expected from injury to the frontal lobe. An ataxic gait would indicate injury primarily to the cerebellum.

Nursing process step: Assessment

Client needs category: Safe, effective care environment

Client needs subcategory: Management of care

Cognitive level: Analysis

---

2. A nurse is assessing a client who reports burning on urination and a low-grade fever. On physical examination, the nurse notes right-sided costovertebral tenderness. Identify the area the nurse percussed to elicit this sign.

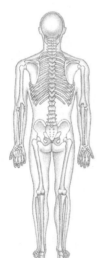

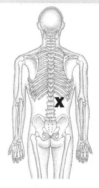
Answer:

Rationale: To determine whether costovertebral tenderness (a sign of glomerulonephritis) is present, the nurse should percuss the costovertebral angle (the angle over each kidney that's formed by the lateral and downward curve of the lowest rib and the vertebral column). The costovertebral angle can be percussed by placing the palm of one hand over the costovertebral angle and striking it with the fist of the other hand.

Nursing process step: Assessment

Client needs category: Physiological integrity

Client needs subcategory: Physiological adaptation

Cognitive level: Application

3. A nurse is assessing a client's abdomen. Identify the area where the nurse's hand should be placed to palpate the liver.

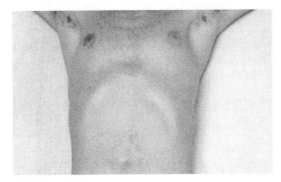

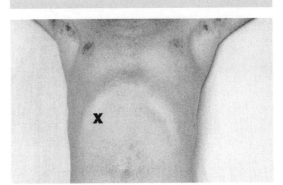

Rationale: The nurse can best palpate the liver by standing on the client's right side and placing her right hand on the client's abdomen, along the right midclavicular line. She should point the fingers of her right hand toward the client's head, just under the right rib margin.

Nursing process step: Assessment

Client needs category: Health promotion and maintenance

Client needs subcategory: None

Cognitive level: Application

---

4. While examining the hands of a client with osteoarthritis, a nurse notes Heberden's nodes on the second (index) finger. Identify the area on the finger where the nurse observed the node.

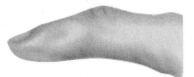

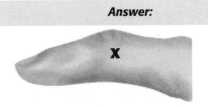

Rationale: Heberden's nodes appear on the distal interphalangeal joints. These bony and cartilaginous enlargements are usually hard and painless and typically occur in middle-aged and elderly clients with osteoarthritis.

Nursing process step: Assessment

Client needs category: Physiological integrity

Client needs subcategory: Physiological adaptation

Cognitive level: Application

5. A nurse is percussing a client's abdomen. Identify the area where liver dullness is best percussed.

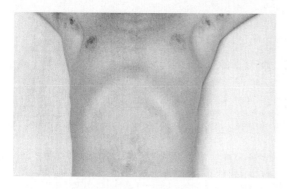

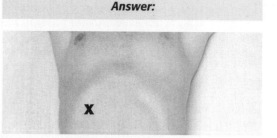

Rationale: To hear liver dullness, the nurse should percuss the abdomen at the right midclavicular line, starting at a level below the umbilicus (in an area of tympany, not dullness) and continuing upward toward the liver.

Nursing process step: Assessment

Client needs category: Health promotion and maintenance

Client needs subcategory: None

Cognitive level: Application

---

6. A client is diagnosed with herpes zoster. Place the pathophysiologic changes associated with the client's disorder in the proper sequence.

1. Fever, malaise, and red nodules appear in dermatome distribution.
2. The virus multiplies in the ganglia, causing deep pain, itching, and paresthesia or hyperesthesia.
3. Vesicles crust and scab but no longer shed the virus.
4. Residual antibodies from the initial infection mobilize but are ineffective.
5. Vesicles appear filled with either clear fluid or pus.
6. Varicella-zoster virus is reactivated.

Answer:

6. Varicella-zoster virus is reactivated.
4. Residual antibodies from the initial infection mobilize but are ineffective.
1. Fever, malaise, and red nodules appear in dermatome distribution.
2. The virus multiplies in the ganglia, causing deep pain, itching, and paresthesia or hyperesthesia.
5. Vesicles appear filled with either clear fluid or pus.
3. Vesicles crust and scab but no longer shed the virus.

Rationale: Herpes zoster is an acute inflammation caused by infection with the herpes virus varicella-zoster (chickenpox virus). The pathophysiologic changes associated with this disorder occur in the order described above.

Nursing process step: Analysis

Client needs category: Physiological integrity

Client needs subcategory: Physiological adaptation

Cognitive level: Application

7. An elderly client has a history of aortic stenosis. Identify the area where the nurse should place the stethoscope to best hear the murmur.

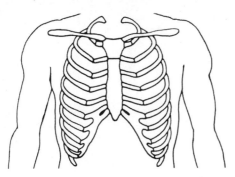

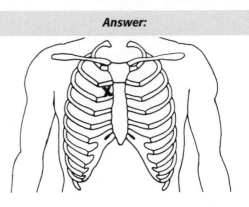

Rationale: The murmur of aortic stenosis is low-pitched, rough, and rasping. It is heard best in the second intercostal space to the right of the sternum.

Nursing process step: Assessment

Client needs category: Physiological integrity

Client needs subcategory: Physiological adaptation

Cognitive level: Application

---

8. A nurse is assessing a client who has a rash on his chest and upper arms. Which questions should the nurse ask in order to gain further information about the client's rash?

Select all that apply.

☐ **1.** "When did the rash start?"

☐ **2.** "Are you allergic to any medications, foods, or pollen?"

☐ **3.** "How old are you?"

☐ **4.** "What have you been using to treat the rash?"

☐ **5.** "Have you recently traveled outside the country?"

☐ **6.** "Do you smoke cigarettes or drink alcohol?"

Answer: 1, 2, 4, 5

Rationale: When assessing a client who has a rash, the nurse should first find out when the rash began; this information can identify where the rash is in the disease process and assist with the correct diagnosis. The nurse should also ask about allergies because rashes related to allergies can occur when a person changes medications, eats new foods, or comes into contact with agents in the air, such as pollen. It's also important for the nurse to find out how the client has been treating the rash because some topical ointments or oral medications may make the rash worse. The nurse should ask about recent travel because travel outside the country exposes the client to foreign foods and environments, which can contribute to the onset of a rash. Although the client's age and smoking and drinking habits can be important to know, this information will not provide further insight into the rash or its cause.

Nursing process step: Assessment

Client needs category: Physiological integrity

Client needs subcategory: Physiological adaptation

Cognitive level: Application

9. While assessing a client's spine for abnormal curvatures, a nurse notes kyphosis. Identify the area of the spine that is affected by kyphosis.

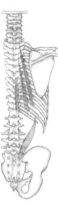

Answer:

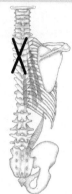

Rationale: Kyphosis is characterized by an accentuated curve of the thoracic area of the spine.

Nursing process step: Assessment

Client needs category: Health promotion and maintenance

Client needs subcategory: None

Cognitive level: Application

---

10. A nurse is auscultating a client's lungs. Identify the area on the client's vertebrae, representing the base of the lungs, where the nurse expects the breath sounds to stop at the end of expiration.

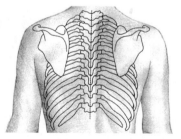

Answer:

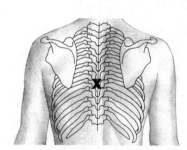

Rationale: Using posterior landmarks, the lungs extend from the cervical area to the level of the 10th thoracic vertebrae (T10) at the end of expiration.

Nursing process step: Assessment

Client needs category: Health promotion and maintenance

Client needs subcategory: None

Cognitive level: Application

11. A nurse is performing an otoscopic examination on a client with ear pain. The nurse notes that the tympanic membrane is bulging and red. Identify the structure that the nurse is assessing.

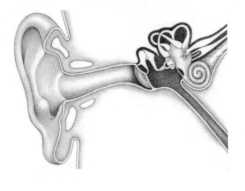

Answer:

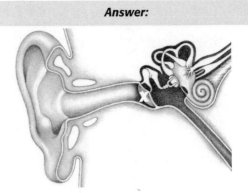

Rationale: The tympanic membrane separates the external and middle ear and may appear red and bulging in a client with otitis media.

Nursing process step: Assessment

Client needs category: Physiological integrity

Client needs subcategory: Physiological adaptation

Cognitive level: Application

---

12. A nurse is performing a cardiac assessment on a client with a suspected murmur. Identify the area where the nurse should place the stethoscope to auscultate Erb's point.

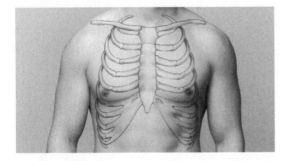

Answer:

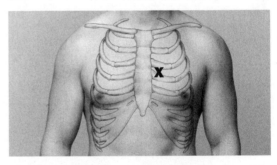

Rationale: Erb's point is located at the third left intercostal space, close to the sternum. Murmurs of both aortic and pulmonic origin may be heard at Erb's point.

Nursing process step: Assessment

Client needs category: Health promotion and maintenance

Client needs subcategory: None

Cognitive level: Application

13. A nurse is performing a head and neck assessment on a client who reports fatigue. Identify the area that the nurse should palpate to assess the occipital lymph nodes.

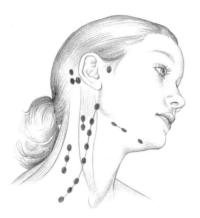

Answer:

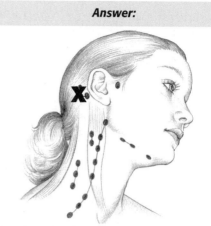

Rationale: Using the pads of the fingers, the nurse should palpate the area behind the ears bilaterally to assess the occipital lymph nodes.

Nursing process step: Assessment

Client needs category: Physiological integrity

Client needs subcategory: Physiological adaptation

Cognitive level: Application

---

14. A nurse is performing a cardiac assessment. Identify the area where the nurse should place the stethoscope to best auscultate the pulmonic valve.

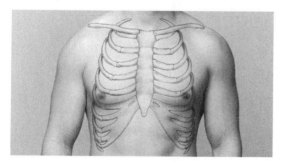

Answer:

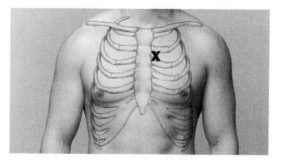

Rationale: The pulmonic valve is best heard at the second intercostal space, just left of the sternum.

Nursing process step: Assessment

Client needs category: Health promotion and maintenance

Client needs subcategory: None

Cognitive level: Application

P A R T **T W O**

Medical-surgical nursing

1. A client with sepsis and hypotension is being treated with dopamine hydrochloride (Inotropin). A nurse asks a colleague to double-check the dosage that the client is receiving. The 250 ml bag contains 400 mg of dopamine, the infusion pump is running at 23 ml/hour, and the client weighs 80 kg. How many micrograms per kilogram per minute is the client receiving?

_____

Answer: 7.7

Rationale: First, calculate how many milligrams per milliliter of dopamine are in the bag:

$$400 \text{ mg}/250 \text{ ml} = 1.6 \text{ mg/ml.}$$

Next, convert milligrams to micrograms:

$$1.6 \text{ mg/ml} \times 1,000 \text{ mcg/mg} = 1,600 \text{ mcg/ml.}$$

Lastly, calculate the dose:

$$\frac{1,600 \text{ mcg}}{1 \text{ ml}} \times \frac{23 \text{ ml}}{60 \text{ minute}} \times \frac{1}{80 \text{ kg}} =$$

$$\frac{36,800 \text{ mcg}}{4,800 \text{ kg/minute}} = 7.7 \text{ mcg/kg/minute.}$$

Nursing process step: Analysis

Client needs category: Physiological integrity

Client needs subcategory: Pharmacological and parenteral therapies

Cognitive level: Analysis

2. A client with deep vein thrombosis is receiving an I.V. infusion of heparin sodium at 1,500 units/hour. The concentration in the bag is 25,000 units/500 ml. How many milliliters should the nurse document as intake from this infusion for an 8-hour shift?

_____

Answer: 240

Rationale: First, calculate how many units are in each milliliter of the medication:

$$25,000 \text{ units}/500 \text{ ml} = 50 \text{ units/ml.}$$

Next, calculate how many milliliters the client receives each hour:

$$1 \text{ ml}/50 \text{ units} \times 1,500 \text{ units/hour} = 30 \text{ ml/hour.}$$

Lastly, multiply by 8 hours:

$$30 \text{ ml/hour} \times 8 \text{ hours} = 240 \text{ ml.}$$

Nursing process step: Analysis

Client needs category: Physiological integrity

Client needs subcategory: Pharmacological and parenteral therapies

Cognitive level: Analysis

3. A nurse is evaluating the following telemetry strips from two of her clients. Based on her review, which of the following statements is true?

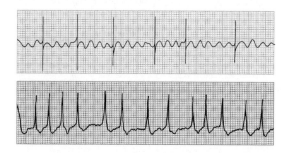

☐ **1.** The ventricular rhythm is irregular in the second strip only.

☐ **2.** The PR interval in the first strip is within the normal range.

☐ **3.** Both strips show atrial abnormalities.

☐ **4.** The second strip shows sawtooth fibrillatory (F) waves.

Rationale: Both clients have atrial abnormalities — the first has atrial flutter, and the second has atrial fibrillation. The ventricular rhythms are irregular in both strips. The PR interval can't be calculated because the strips show no clear-cut P waves, just F waves of varied intensity in each. The first strip shows the sawtooth pattern of F waves characteristic of lead II in atrial flutter.

Nursing process step: Analysis

Client needs category: Physiological integrity

Client needs subcategory: Physiological adaptation

Cognitive level: Application

---

4. A nurse is interpreting a client's telemetry strip. If the PR interval measures four small blocks, how many seconds is the PR interval?

_____

Rationale: Each small block on a telemetry strip graph represents 0.04 second. So multiply as follows:

4 blocks × 0.04 second = 0.16 second.

Nursing process step: Analysis

Client needs category: Physiological integrity

Client needs subcategory: Reduction of risk potential

Cognitive level: Application

5. A nurse is caring for a client with Raynaud's phenomenon secondary to systemic lupus erythematosus. Which of the following client statements shows an understanding of the nurse's teaching about this disorder?

Select all that apply.

☐ **1.** "My hands get pale, bluish, and feel numb and painful when I'm really stressed."

☐ **2.** "I can't continue to wash dishes and do my cleaning because of this problem."

☐ **3.** "I don't need to report any other skin problems with my fingers or hands to my primary care provider."

☐ **4.** "I probably got this disorder because I have lupus."

☐ **5.** "This problem is caused by a temporary lack of circulation in my hands."

☐ **6.** "Medication might help treat this problem."

Answer: 1, 4, 5, 6

Rationale: Raynaud's phenomenon causes blanching, cyanosis, coldness, numbness, and throbbing pain in the hands when the client is exposed to cold or stress. It's caused by episodic vasospasm in the small peripheral arteries and arterioles and can affect the feet as well as the hands. The phenomenon is commonly associated with connective tissue diseases such as lupus and may be alleviated by calcium channel blockers or adrenergic blockers. It doesn't limit the client's ability to function, although the symptoms are bothersome. Keeping the hands warm and learning to manage stressful situations effectively reduces the frequency of episodes. The disorder can progress to skin ulcerations and even gangrene in some clients, so all skin changes should be reported to the primary care provider promptly.

Nursing process step: Evaluation

Client needs category: Physiological integrity

Client needs subcategory: Physiological adaptation

Cognitive level: Analysis

---

6. A nurse is evaluating the 12-lead electrocardiogram (ECG) of a client experiencing an inferior wall myocardial infarction (MI). While conferring with the team, she correctly identifies which of the following ECG changes associated with an evolving MI?

Select all that apply.

☐ **1.** Notched T wave

☐ **2.** Presence of a U wave

☐ **3.** T-wave inversion

☐ **4.** Prolonged PR interval

☐ **5.** ST-segment elevation

☐ **6.** Pathologic Q wave

Answer: 3, 5, 6

Rationale: T-wave inversion, ST-segment elevation, and a pathologic Q wave are all signs of tissue hypoxia that occur during an MI. Ischemia results from inadequate blood supply to the myocardial tissue and is reflected by T-wave inversion. Injury results from prolonged ischemia and is reflected by ST-segment elevation. Q waves may become evident when the injury progresses to infarction. A notched T wave may indicate pericarditis in an adult client. A U wave may be apparent on a normal ECG; it represents repolarization of the Purkinje fibers. A prolonged PR interval is associated with first-degree atrioventricular block.

Nursing process step: Evaluation

Client needs category: Physiological integrity

Client needs subcategory: Physiological adaptation

Cognitive level: Analysis

7. A client with a bicuspid aortic valve has severe stenosis and is scheduled for valve replacement. While teaching the client about his condition and upcoming surgery, a nurse shows him a heart illustration. Identify the valve that the nurse should indicate will be replaced.

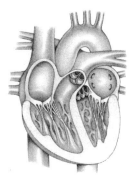

Answer:

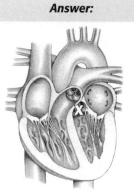

Rationale: The aortic valve is located between the left ventricle and the aorta. It's one of the semilunar valves and normally has three cusps. A person with a bicuspid aortic valve is at risk for aortic stenosis and aortic regurgitation. This impaired blood flow through the valve leads to increased pumping pressure of the left ventricle.

Nursing process step: Planning

Client needs category: Physiological integrity

Client needs subcategory: Physiological adaptation

Cognitive level: Application

---

8. A nurse is awaiting the arrival of a client from the emergency department who is being admitted with a left ventricular myocardial infarction. In caring for this client, the nurse should be alert for which of the following signs and symptoms of left-sided heart failure?

Select all that apply.

☐ **1.** Jugular vein distention

☐ **2.** Hepatomegaly

☐ **3.** Dyspnea

☐ **4.** Crackles

☐ **5.** Tachycardia

☐ **6.** Right-upper-quadrant pain

Answer: 3, 4, 5

Rationale: Signs and symptoms of left-sided heart failure include dyspnea, orthopnea, and paroxysmal nocturnal dyspnea; fatigue; nonproductive cough and crackles; hemoptysis; point of maximal impulse displaced toward the left anterior axillary line; tachycardia; S_3 and S_4 heart sounds; and cool, pale skin. Jugular vein distention, hepatomegaly, and right-upper-quadrant pain are all signs of right-sided heart failure.

Nursing process step: Assessment

Client needs category: Physiological integrity

Client needs subcategory: Physiological adaptation

Cognitive level: Application

9. A client is admitted to the emergency department after complaining of acute chest pain radiating down his left arm. Which of the following laboratory studies would be indicated?

Select all that apply.

☐ **1.** Hemoglobin and hematocrit

☐ **2.** Serum glucose

☐ **3.** Creatine kinase (CK)

☐ **4.** Troponin T and troponin I

☐ **5.** Myoglobin

☐ **6.** Blood urea nitrogen (BUN)

Answer: 3, 4, 5

Rationale: Levels of CK, troponin T, and troponin I would rise because of cellular damage. Myoglobin elevation is an early indicator of myocardial damage. Hemoglobin, hematocrit, serum glucose, and BUN levels don't provide information related to myocardial ischemia.

Nursing process step: Planning

Client needs category: Health promotion and maintenance

Client needs subcategory: None

Cognitive level: Application

---

10. A client is prescribed lisinopril (Zestril) for treatment of hypertension. He asks a nurse about possible adverse effects. The nurse should teach him about which of the following common adverse effects of angiotensin-converting enzyme (ACE) inhibitors?

Select all that apply.

☐ **1.** Constipation

☐ **2.** Dizziness

☐ **3.** Headache

☐ **4.** Hyperglycemia

☐ **5.** Hypotension

☐ **6.** Impotence

Answer: 2, 3, 5

Rationale: Dizziness, headache, and hypotension are all common adverse effects of lisinopril and other ACE inhibitors. Lisinopril may cause diarrhea, not constipation. Lisinopril isn't known to cause hyperglycemia or impotence.

Nursing process step: Implementation

Client needs category: Physiological integrity

Client needs subcategory: Pharmacological and parenteral therapies

Cognitive level: Application

11. A nurse is performing a 12-lead electrocardiogram (ECG) on a client who's complaining of chest pain. Identify the area where lead V_6 should be placed.

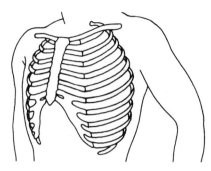

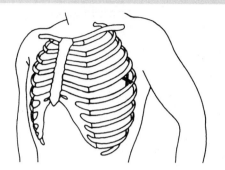

Rationale: The V_6 lead should be placed at the fifth intercostal space at the midaxillary line. Correct placement of the leads is essential when performing a 12-lead ECG to accurately document the electrical potential of the heart. V_6 is one of the precordial leads and, in combination with the other leads, records potential in the horizontal plane.

Nursing process step: Implementation

Client needs category: Physiological integrity

Client needs subcategory: Reduction of risk potential

Cognitive level: Application

---

12. A nurse is counseling a client about risk factors for hypertension. Which of the following should the nurse list as risk factors for primary hypertension?

Select all that apply.

☐ **1.** Obesity

☐ **2.** Glomerulonephritis

☐ **3.** Head injury

☐ **4.** Stress

☐ **5.** Hormonal contraceptive use

☐ **6.** High intake of sodium or saturated fat

Answer: 1, 4, 6

Rationale: Obesity, stress, high intake of sodium or saturated fat, and family history are all risk factors for primary hypertension. Diabetes mellitus, head injury, and hormonal contraceptive use are risk factors for secondary hypertension.

Nursing process step: Assessment

Client needs category: Health promotion and maintenance

Client needs subcategory: None

Cognitive level: Application

13. A nurse is caring for a client with first-degree atrioventricular (AV) block. Identify the area in the conduction cycle of the heart where this block occurs.

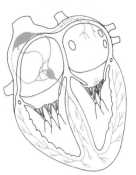

Answer:

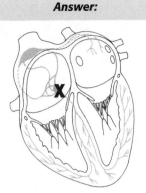

Rationale: First-degree AV block is a conduction disturbance in which electrical impulses flow normally from the sinoatrial node through the atria but are delayed at the AV node.

Nursing process step: Assessment

Client needs category: Physiological integrity

Client needs subcategory: Physiological adaptation

Cognitive level: Analysis

Oncologic disorders

1. A client in the terminal stage of cancer is being transferred to hospice care. Which information regarding hospice care should the nurse include in the teaching plan?

Select all that apply.

☐ **1.** The focus of care is on controlling symptoms and relieving pain.

☐ **2.** A multidisciplinary team provides care.

☐ **3.** Services are provided based on the ability to pay.

☐ **4.** Hospice care is provided only in hospice centers.

☐ **5.** Bereavement care is provided to the family.

☐ **6.** Care is provided in the home, independent of physicians.

Answer: 1, 2, 5

Rationale: Hospice care focuses on controlling symptoms and relieving pain at the end of life. A multidisciplinary team — consisting of nurses, physicians, chaplains, aides, and volunteers — provides the care. After the client's death, hospice provides bereavement care to the grieving family. Hospice services are provided based on need, not on the ability to pay. Hospice care may be provided in a variety of settings, such as free-standing hospice centers, the home, a hospital, or a long-term care facility. Care is provided under the direction of a physician, who's a key member of the hospice team.

Nursing process step: Planning

Client needs category: Physiological integrity

Client needs subcategory: Basic care and comfort

Cognitive level: Application

2. An adult client with Hodgkin's disease who weighs 143 lb is to receive vincristine (Oncovin) 25 mcg/kg I.V. What is the correct dose in micrograms that the client should receive?

_____

Answer: 1625

Rationale: First, convert the client's weight from pounds to kilograms:

$$1 \text{ lb} = 2.2 \text{ kg}$$

$$143 \text{ lb} = X \text{ kg}$$

$$143 \text{ lb}/2.2 \text{ kg} = 65 \text{ kg}.$$

Next, multiply the weight in kilograms by the number of micrograms desired per kilogram:

$$65 \text{ kg} \times 25 \text{ mcg} = 1,625 \text{ mcg}.$$

Nursing process step: Implementation

Client needs category: Physiological integrity

Client needs subcategory: Pharmacological and parenteral therapies

Cognitive level: Application

---

3. A nurse has identified the nursing diagnosis _Situational low self-esteem related to hair loss and severe fatigue_ in a client with cancer. Which of the following nursing interventions would be appropriate for this client's care?

Select all that apply.

☐ **1.** Ask the client how the diagnosis and treatment are affecting her personal life and roles.

☐ **2.** Review any anticipated side effects of treatment with the client, stressing that some may not occur and others can be controlled.

☐ **3.** Teach the client how to solve specific concerns related to the effects of treatment on her personal life.

☐ **4.** As a guide for behavior, describe the experiences of friends and other clients who have had this disease and treatment.

☐ **5.** Offer information on available counseling services and support groups, if desired, explaining that these techniques are helpful to many clients.

☐ **6.** Use touch during interactions, if acceptable to the client, and maintain eye contact during interactions.

Answer: 1, 2, 5, 6

Rationale: Discussing the client's feelings about her cancer diagnosis and treatment help to identify coping-related problems. Anticipating potential adverse effects can help the client begin to adapt and prepare to cope with these events. Referral to support groups or counseling services helps provide the client with validation and assistance with problem solving. Touch and eye contact can be therapeutic in affirming individuality and acceptance and can help build self-esteem. Instructing the client in how the nurse believes problems should be resolved isn't therapeutic. The nurse should help the client explore options for solving her problems in a manner consistent with the client's beliefs and values. Telling stories about others' experiences without their consent breaches the right to privacy and may demonstrate a lack of listening and empathetic interaction by the nurse. Validating the client's own personal story is beneficial to rebuilding self esteem.

Nursing process step: Planning

Client needs category: Psychosocial integrity

Client needs subcategory: None

Cognitive level: Analysis

4. A client with laryngeal cancer has undergone a laryngectomy and is now receiving radiation therapy to the head and neck. The nurse should monitor the client for which of the following adverse effects of external radiation?

Select all that apply.

☐ **1.** Xerostomia

☐ **2.** Stomatitis

☐ **3.** Thrombocytopenia

☐ **4.** Cystitis

☐ **5.** Dysgeusia

☐ **6.** Leukopenia

Answer: 1, 2, 5

Rationale: Radiation of the head and neck often produces dry mouth (xerostomia), irritation of the oral mucous membranes (stomatitis), and diminished sense of taste (dysgeusia). Thrombocytopenia (reduced platelet count) and leukopenia (reduced white blood cell count) may occur with systemic radiation; cystitis may occur with radiation of the genitourinary system.

Nursing process step: Assessment

Client needs category: Physiological integrity

Client needs subcategory: Reduction of risk potential

Cognitive level: Application

---

5. A nurse is teaching a community program on breast self-examination. She teaches the clients the proper procedure for palpating each breast. In what sequence should the following actions be performed for proper self-examination?

1. Use the right hand for the left breast and vice versa.
2. Lie down with an arm behind the head.
3. Palpate the breast in a perpendicular motion, going across the breast from side to side and top to bottom.
4. Use a circular motion to feel the breast tissue (with light, medium, and firm pressure).
5. Use the finger pads of the three middle fingers.

Answer:

2. Lie down with an arm behind the head.
1. Use the right hand for the left breast and vice versa.
5. Use the finger pads of the three middle fingers.
4. Use a circular motion to feel the breast tissue (with light, medium, and firm pressure).
3. Palpate the breast in a perpendicular motion, going across the breast from side to side and top to bottom.

Rationale: Breast self-examination is a standard procedure described by national organizations designed to ensure palpation of all breast tissue. The exam also includes a visual inspection of the breasts while pressing the hands firmly against the hips and examining the underarms of each breast with arms slightly raised.

Nursing process step: Implementation

Client needs category: Health promotion and maintenance

Client needs subcategory: None

Cognitive level: Application

6. A client who is receiving chemotherapy for breast cancer develops myelosuppression. Which of the following instructions should a nurse include in the client's discharge teaching plan?

Select all that apply.

☐ **1.** Avoid people who have recently received vaccines.

☐ **2.** Avoid activities that may cause bleeding.

☐ **3.** Wash hands frequently.

☐ **4.** Increase intake of fresh fruits and vegetables.

☐ **5.** Avoid crowded places such as shopping malls.

☐ **6.** Treat a sore throat with over-the-counter products.

Answer: 1, 2, 3, 5

Rationale: Chemotherapy can cause myelosuppression, which is a deceased number of red blood cells, white blood cells, and platelets. A client receiving chemotherapy needs to avoid people who have been vaccinated recently because an exaggerated reaction may occur. Because platelet counts are reduced, the client also needs to avoid activities that could cause trauma and bleeding. The client should wash her hands frequently because hand washing is the best way to prevent the spread of infection. A client receiving chemotherapy should avoid crowded places as well as people with colds during the flu season because she has a reduced ability to fight infection. Fresh fruits and vegetables should be avoided because they can harbor bacteria that can't be removed easily by washing. Signs and symptoms of infection, such as a sore throat, fever, and a cough, should be reported immediately to the primary care provider.

Nursing process step: Planning

Client needs category: Physiological integrity

Client needs subcategory: Reduction of risk potential

Cognitive level: Application

---

7. A client with bladder cancer undergoes surgical removal of the bladder with construction of an ileal conduit. Which assessment findings by the nurse indicate that the client is developing complications?

Select all that apply.

☐ **1.** Urine output greater than 30 ml/hour

☐ **2.** Dusky appearance of the stoma

☐ **3.** Stoma protrusion from the skin

☐ **4.** Mucus shreds in the urine collection bag

☐ **5.** Edema of the stoma during the first 24 hours after surgery

☐ **6.** Sharp abdominal pain with rigidity

Answer: 2, 3, 6

Rationale: A dusky appearance of the stoma indicates decreased blood supply; a healthy stoma should appear beefy-red. Protrusion indicates prolapse of the stoma, and sharp abdominal pain with rigidity suggests peritonitis. A urine output greater than 30 ml/hour is a sign of adequate renal perfusion and is a normal finding. Because mucous membranes are used to create the conduit, mucus in the urine is expected. Stomal edema is a normal finding during the first 24 hours after surgery.

Nursing process step: Assessment

Client needs category: Physiological integrity

Client needs subcategory: Reduction of risk potential

Cognitive level: Analysis

ONCOLOGIC DISORDERS **37**

8. A client is ordered a dose of epoetin alfa to treat anemia related to chemotherapy. The recommended dose is 150 units/kg. The client weighs 60 kg. The vial is labeled 10,000 units/ml. The nurse should administer how many milliliters of epoetin alfa?

_____

Answer: 0.9

Rationale: First determine the number of units of epoetin alfa the client is to receive:

$$60 \text{ kg} \times 150 \text{ units} = 9000 \text{ units/kg.}$$

Next, determine the number of milliliters required to deliver that dose:

$$10,000 \text{ units} : 1 \text{ ml} = 9000 \text{ units} : X$$

$$10,000X = 9000$$

$$X = 0.9 \text{ ml.}$$

Nursing process step: Planning

Client needs category: Physiological Integrity

Client needs subcategory: Pharmacological and parenteral therapies

Cognitive level: Application

Gastrointestinal disorders

1. A nurse is reviewing the causes of gastro-esophageal reflux disease (GERD) with a client. What area of the GI tract should the nurse identify as the cause of reduced pressure associated with GERD?

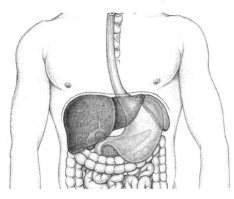

Answer:

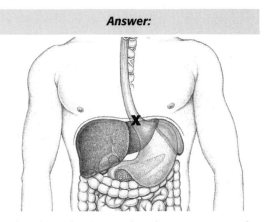

Rationale: Reflux occurs when the pressure around the cardiac or lower esophageal sphincter (LES) is deficient or when pressure in the stomach exceeds LES pressure.

Nursing process step: Implementation

Client needs category: Health promotion and maintenance

Client needs subcategory: None

Cognitive level: Application

2. As part of a routine screening for colorectal cancer, a client must undergo fecal occult blood testing. Which foods should the nurse instruct the client to avoid for 48 to 72 hours before the test and throughout the collection period?

Select all that apply.

☐ **1.** High-fiber foods

☐ **2.** Red meat

☐ **3.** Turnips

☐ **4.** Cantaloupe

☐ **5.** Tomatoes

☐ **6.** Peas

Answer: 2, 3, 4

Rationale: The client should avoid red meat, poultry, and fish as well as beets, broccoli, cauliflower, horseradish, mushrooms, and turnips. Such fruits as cantaloupe, melons, and grapefruit also are prohibited. Tomatoes and peas are acceptable. The client should be taught to maintain a high-fiber diet in order to promote colonic emptying time and fecal bulk, which aid in obtaining specimens.

Nursing process step: Implementation

Client needs category: Health promotion and maintenance

Client needs subcategory: None

Cognitive level: Application

---

3. A client returns from the operating room after undergoing extensive abdominal surgery. He is receiving 1,000 ml of lactated Ringer's solution via a central line infusion. The primary care provider orders the I.V. fluid to be infused at 125 ml/hour plus the total output of the previous hour. The drip factor of the tubing is 15 gtt/ml and the output for the previous hour was 75 ml via Foley catheter, 50 ml via nasogastric tube, and 10 ml via Jackson Pratt tube. For how many drops (gtt) per minute should the nurse set the I.V. flow rate to deliver the correct amount of fluid?

_____

Answer: 65

Rationale: First, calculate the volume to be infused (in milliliters):

$$75 \text{ ml} + 50 \text{ ml} + 10 \text{ ml} =$$
$$135 \text{ ml total output for the previous hour}$$

$$135 \text{ ml} + 125 \text{ ml ordered as a constant flow} =$$
$$260 \text{ ml to be infused over the next hour.}$$

Next, use the formula:

$$\text{Volume to be infused/Total minutes}$$
$$\text{to be infused} \times \text{Drip factor} = \text{Drops per minute.}$$

In this case:

$$260 \text{ ml} \div 60 \text{ minutes} \times 15 \text{ gtt/ml} =$$
$$65 \text{ gtt/minute.}$$

Nursing process step: Implementation

Client needs category: Physiological integrity

Client needs subcategory: Pharmacological and parenteral therapies

Cognitive level: Analysis

4. A client with a retroperitoneal abscess is receiving gentamicin (Garamycin). Which of the following should the nurse monitor?

Select all that apply.

☐ **1.** Hearing

☐ **2.** Urine output

☐ **3.** Hematocrit (HCT)

☐ **4.** Blood urea nitrogen (BUN) and serum creatinine levels

☐ **5.** Serum calcium level

Answer: 1, 2, 4

Rationale: Adverse effects of gentamicin include ototoxicity and nephrotoxicity. The nurse must monitor the client's hearing and instruct him to report any hearing loss or tinnitus. Signs of nephrotoxicity include decreased urine output and elevated BUN and serum creatinine levels. Gentamicin doesn't affect the serum calcium level or HCT.

Nursing process step: Assessment

Client needs category: Physiological integrity

Client needs subcategory: Pharmacological and parenteral therapies

Cognitive level: Analysis

---

5. A nurse is assessing the abdomen of a client who was admitted to the emergency department with suspected appendicitis. Identify the area of the abdomen that the nurse should palpate last.

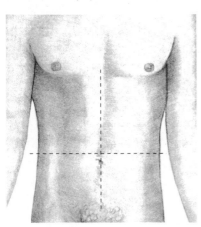

Answer:

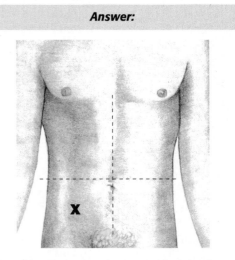

Rationale: An acute attack of appendicitis localizes as pain and tenderness in the lower right quadrant, midway between the umbilicus and the crest of the ilium. This area should be palpated last in order to determine if pain is also present in other areas of the abdomen.

Nursing process step: Assessment

Client needs category: Physiological integrity

Client needs subcategory: Physiological adaptation

Cognitive level: Application

6. While preparing a client for an upper GI endoscopy (esophagogastroduodenoscopy), a nurse should implement which of the following interventions?

Select all that apply.

- ☐ **1.** Administer a preparation to cleanse the GI tract, such as Golytely or Fleets Phospha-Soda.
- ☐ **2.** Tell the client he shouldn't eat or drink for 6 to 12 hours before the procedure.
- ☐ **3.** Tell the client he must be on a clear liquid diet for 24 hours before the procedure.
- ☐ **4.** Inform the client that he'll receive a sedative before the procedure.
- ☐ **5.** Tell the client that he may eat and drink immediately after the procedure.

Answer: 2, 4

Rationale: The client shouldn't eat or drink for 6 to 12 hours before the procedure to ensure that his upper GI tract is clear for viewing. Before the endoscope is inserted, the client will receive a sedative that will help him relax, but leave him conscious. GI tract cleansing and a clear liquid diet are interventions for a client having a lower GI tract procedure, such as a colonoscopy. Food and fluids must be withheld until the gag reflex returns after the procedure.

Nursing process step: Implementation

Client needs category: Physiological integrity

Client needs subcategory: Reduction of risk potential

Cognitive level: Application

---

7. A nurse is caring for a client who recently had a bowel resection. The client has a hemoglobin level of 8 g/dl and hematocrit of 30%. Dextrose 5% in half-normal saline solution ($D_5\frac{1}{2}NS$) is infusing through a triple-lumen central catheter at 125 ml/hour. The primary care provider's orders include:

- gentamicin (Garamycin) 80 mg I.V. piggyback in 50 ml dextrose 5% in water (D_5W) over 30 minutes
- ranitidine (Zantac) 50 mg I.V. in 50 ml D_5W piggyback over 30 minutes
- one unit of 250 ml of packed red blood cells (RBCs) over 3 hours
- nasogastric tube flushes with 30 ml normal saline solution every 2 hours.

How many milliliters should the nurse document as the total intake for the 8-hour shift?

_____

Answer: 1470

Rationale: Add up the total intake as follows:

- regular I.V. of $D_5\frac{1}{2}NS$ at 125 ml $\times$ 8 hours = 1,000 ml
- gentamicin piggyback = 50 ml
- ranitidine piggyback = 50 ml
- packed RBCs = 250 ml
- nasogastric flushes 30 ml $\times$ 4 = 120 ml
- total = 1,470 ml.

Nursing process step: Implementation

Client needs category: Physiological integrity

Client needs subcategory: Physiological adaptation

Cognitive level: Analysis

8. Indicate the location of an ostomy for which a client might eventually not need to wear an ostomy bag?

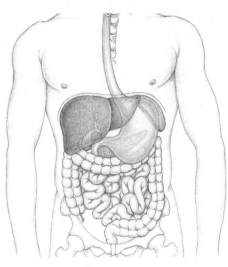

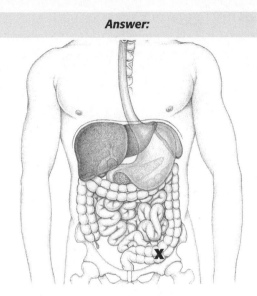

Rationale: With a sigmoid colostomy, the feces are solid; therefore, the client might eventually gain enough control that he would not need to wear a colostomy bag. With a descending colostomy, the feces are semi-soft. With a transverse colostomy, the feces are soft. With an ascending colostomy, the feces are fluid. In these three latter cases, the client would be unlikely to gain control of elimination and consequently would need to continue wearing an ostomy bag.

Nursing process step: Planning

Client needs category: Physiological integrity

Client needs subcategory: Basic care and comfort

Cognitive level: Application

---

9. Which of the following findings are common in clients with acute diverticulitis?

Select all that apply.

☐ **1.** Vomiting

☐ **2.** Cramping pain in the left lower abdominal quadrant

☐ **3.** Bowel irregularity

☐ **4.** Heartburn

☐ **5.** Intervals of diarrhea

☐ **6.** Hiccuping

Answer: 2, 3, 5

Rationale: Signs and symptoms of acute diverticulitis include bowel irregularity, intervals of diarrhea, abrupt onset of cramping pain in the left lower abdomen, and a low-grade fever. Vomiting, heartburn, and hiccuping are not signs of acute diverticulitis.

Nursing process step: Assessment

Client needs category: Physiological integrity

Client needs subcategory: Physiological adaptation

Cognitive level: Analysis

10. A 28-year-old client is admitted with inflammatory bowel syndrome (Crohn's disease). Which of the following should a nurse expect to be part of the care plan?

Select all that apply.

☐ **1.** Lactulose therapy

☐ **2.** High-fiber diet

☐ **3.** High-protein milkshakes

☐ **4.** Corticosteroid therapy

☐ **5.** Antidiarrheal medications

Rationale: Corticosteroids, such as prednisone, reduce the signs and symptoms of diarrhea, pain, and bleeding by decreasing inflammation. Antidiarrheals, such as diphenoxylate (Lomotil), combat diarrhea by decreasing peristalsis. Lactulose is used to treat chronic constipation and would aggravate the symptoms of Crohn's disease. A high-fiber diet and milk and milk products are contraindicated in clients with Crohn's disease because they may promote diarrhea.

Nursing process step: Planning

Client needs category: Safe, effective care environment

Client needs subcategory: Management of care

Cognitive level: Analysis

Integumentary disorders

1. A 30-year-old presents at the physician's office with gray-brown burrows with epidermal curved ridges and follicular papules of the skin. The primary care provider diagnoses scabies. Which of the following teaching points should a nurse review with the client?

Select all that apply.

☐ **1.** The disease is only actively contagious when the lesions are open.

☐ **2.** Scabies is transmitted by close person-to-person contact or contact with infected linens and clothing.

☐ **3.** The most commonly infected areas are the hands, feet, and neck.

☐ **4.** Severe itching of the affected areas, especially at night, is a common finding.

☐ **5.** Only the infected individual needs to use the prescribed medication.

☐ **6.** All of the client's linens and clothing should immediately be washed in hot water.

Rationale: Scabies is a contagious disorder caused by a tiny mite that burrows under the skin; it's transmitted by close person-to-person contact or contact with infected linens or clothing. It causes severe itching, especially at night, in addition to the familiar papular rash. All of the client's linens and clothing should be washed promptly to reduce the risk of reinfestation. Scabies is transmissible from the time of infection to the time the burrows and papules appear, which may occur several weeks afterward. It remains transmissible until eradicated by a prescription cream or an oral medication. Scabies is most commonly seen in the finger webs, flexor surface of the wrists, and the antecubital fossae. When a family member is diagnosed, all members of the family must be treated with medication and their clothing and linens washed to prevent transmission and reinfestation.

Nursing process step: Planning

Client needs category: Health promotion and maintenance

Client needs subcategory: None

Cognitive level: Application

2. At an outpatient clinic, a medical assistant interviews a client and documents her findings, as follows:

12/13/05	Client very anxious because new black mole
0900	with shades of brown noted on upper outer
	right thigh. Asymmetrical in shape with an
	irregular border.————M. Rosenfeld, MA

After reading the chart note, a nurse begins planning based on which of the following nursing diagnoses?

☐ **1.** Deficient knowledge related to potential diagnosis of basal cell carcinoma

☐ **2.** Fear related to potential diagnosis of malignant melanoma

☐ **3.** Risk for impaired skin integrity related to potential squamous cell carcinoma

☐ **4.** Readiness for enhanced knowledge of skin care precautions related to benign mole

---

Answer: 2

Rationale: Documentation reveals that the client is anxious about her symptoms. These symptoms (asymmetry, variable color, and border irregularity) most closely resemble malignant melanoma. Therefore, *Fear related to potential diagnosis of malignant melanoma* is the most appropriate nursing diagnosis. The nursing note contains no indication that the client presently has deficient knowledge. The characteristics of the lesion are not consistent with basal or squamous cell carcinoma or a benign nevus (mole).

Nursing process step: Analysis

Client needs category: Physiological integrity

Client needs subcategory: Physiological adaptation

Cognitive level: Analysis

---

3. While assessing a client with a stage 2 pressure ulcer, a nurse observes which of the following criteria?

Select all that apply.

☐ **1.** The skin is intact.

☐ **2.** Full-thickness skin loss is evident.

☐ **3.** Undermining is present.

☐ **4.** Sinus tracts have developed.

☐ **5.** The ulcer is superficial like a blister.

☐ **6.** Partial-thickness skin loss of the epidermis is evident.

Answer: 5, 6

Rationale: A stage 2 pressure ulcer involves partial-thickness skin loss of the epidermis or dermis. The ulcer is superficial and presents clinically as an abrasion, blister, or shallow crater. Intact skin is a characteristic of a stage 1 pressure ulcer. Full-thickness skin loss, undermining, and sinus tracts are characteristics of a stage 3 pressure ulcer.

Nursing process step: Assessment

Client needs category: Physiological integrity

Client needs subcategory: Physiological adaptation

Cognitive level: Analysis

4. A nurse is planning the care for a client with a pressure ulcer. Which of the following statements should the nurse include in the client's nursing care plan?

Select all that apply.

☐ **1.** Use pressure reduction devices.

☐ **2.** Increase carbohydrates in the diet.

☐ **3.** Reposition the client every 1 to 2 hours.

☐ **4.** Teach the family how to care for the wound.

☐ **5.** Clean the area around the ulcer with mild soap.

☐ **6.** Avoid the use of support-surface therapy.

Answer: 1, 3, 4, 5

Rationale: Using a pressure reduction device, repositioning the client every 1 to 2 hours, and cleaning the area around the wound with a mild soap will aid in healing or prevent further skin breakdown. Teaching the family how to care for the wound will assist with discharge planning. Protein, not carbohydrate, intake, should be increased to promote wound healing. Support-surface therapy is a major therapeutic method of managing pressure, friction, and shear on tissues.

Nursing process step: Planning

Client needs category: Physiological integrity

Client needs subcategory: Basic care and comfort

Cognitive level: Analysis

---

5. A triage nurse in the emergency department admits a 50-year-old male client with second-degree burns on the anterior and posterior portions of both legs. Based on the Rule of Nines, what percentage of the body is burned?

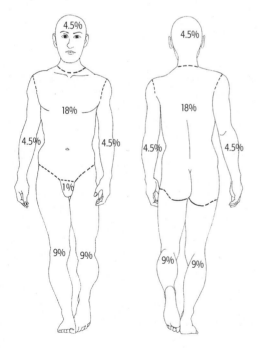

Answer: 36

Rationale: The anterior and posterior portions of one leg amount to 18%. Because both legs are burned, the total is 36%.

Nursing process step: Assessment

Client needs category: Physiological integrity

Client needs subcategory: Physiological adaptation

Cognitive level: Analysis

6. A client returns from the operating room with a partial-thickness skin graft on her left arm. The donor tissue was taken from her left hip. In planning her immediate postoperative care, which of the following interventions should the nurse include?

Select all that apply.

☐ **1.** Change the dressing on the graft site every 8 hours.

☐ **2.** Elevate the left arm and provide complete rest of the grafted area.

☐ **3.** Administer pain medication every 4 hours as ordered for pain in donor site.

☐ **4.** Perform range-of-motion (ROM) exercises to the left arm every 4 hours.

☐ **5.** Monitor the pulse in the left arm every 4 hours.

☐ **6.** Encourage the client to ambulate as desired on the first postoperative day.

Answer: 2, 3, 5

Rationale: The left arm should be elevated to reduce edema. Complete rest of the arm is needed to allow the graft to adhere. The donor site is usually more painful than the graft site, and the client will require pain medication to obtain relief. Because adequate circulation is needed for graft healing, it's important to monitor for pulse presence. Changing the dressing every 8 hours, performing ROM exercises every 4 hours, and ambulating on the first day are inappropriate because postoperative graft sites require immobilization for 3 to 5 days.

Nursing process step: Planning

Client needs category: Physiological integrity

Client needs subcategory: Physiological adaptation

Cognitive level: Application

Immune and hematologic disorders

1. A nurse is preparing a client with systemic lupus erythematosus (SLE) for discharge. Which instructions should the nurse include in the teaching plan?

Select all that apply.

☐ **1.** Stay out of direct sunlight.

☐ **2.** Don't limit activity between flare-ups.

☐ **3.** Monitor body temperature.

☐ **4.** Taper the corticosteroid dosage as prescribed when symptoms are under control.

☐ **5.** Apply cold packs to relieve joint pain and stiffness.

Answer: 1, 3, 4

Rationale: A client with SLE should stay out of direct sunlight and avoid other sources of ultraviolet light because they may trigger severe skin reactions and exacerbate the symptoms. The client's body temperature should be monitored and fevers reported to the primary health care provider. The corticosteroid dosage must be tapered gradually once symptoms are relieved because stopping these drugs abruptly can cause adrenal insufficiency, a potentially life-threatening condition. Fatigue can cause an SLE flare-up, so the client should pace activities and plan for rest periods. The client should apply heat, not cold, to relieve joint pain. Cold packs may aggravate Raynaud's phenomenon, which commonly occurs in clients with SLE.

Nursing process step: Planning

Client needs category: Physiological integrity

Client needs subcategory: Reduction of risk potential

Cognitive level: Application

2. A client is to receive a blood transfusion of packed red blood cells for severe anemia. Place the following steps in the order a nurse would follow to administer this product.

1. Flush the I.V. tubing and line with normal saline solution.

2. Verify the blood bag identification, ABO group, and Rh compatibility against the client information.

3. Remain with the client and watch for signs of a transfusion reaction.

4. Record vital signs.

5. Put on gloves, a gown, and a face shield.

6. Check the packed cells for abnormal color, clumping, gas bubbles, and expiration date.

4. Record vital signs.

6. Check the packed cells for abnormal color, clumping, gas bubbles, and expiration date.

2. Verify the blood bag identification, ABO group, and Rh compatibility against the client information.

5. Put on gloves, a gown, and a face shield.

1. Flush the I.V. tubing and line with normal saline solution.

3. Remain with the client and watch for signs of a transfusion reaction.

Rationale: To administer a blood transfusion, the nurse should follow the steps listed above. Note that the transfusion may be withheld if the client's temperature is 100° F or greater. Two client identifiers must be checked before the transfusion.

Nursing process step: Implementation

Client needs category: Physiological integrity

Client needs subcategory: Pharmacological and parenteral therapies

Cognitive level: Application

---

3. A nurse is planning care for a client with human immunodeficiency virus (HIV) infection. She's being assisted by a licensed practical nurse (LPN). Which statements by the LPN indicate her understanding of HIV transmission?

Select all that apply.

☐ **1.** "I'll wear a gown, mask, and gloves for all client contact."

☐ **2.** "I don't need to wear any personal protective equipment because nurses have a low risk of occupational exposure."

☐ **3.** "I'll wear a mask if the client has a cough caused by an upper respiratory infection."

☐ **4.** "I'll wear a mask, gown, and gloves when splashing of body fluids is likely."

☐ **5.** "I'll wash my hands after client care."

Answer: 4, 5

Rationale: Standard precautions include wearing gloves for any known or anticipated contact with blood, body fluids, tissue, mucous membranes, or nonintact skin. If the task may result in splashing or splattering of blood or body fluids, a mask and goggles or a face shield and a fluid-resistant gown or apron should be worn. Hands should be washed before and after client care and after removing gloves.

Nursing process step: Planning

Client needs category: Safe, effective care environment

Client needs subcategory: Safety and infection control

Cognitive level: Comprehension

4. Which nonpharmacologic interventions should a nurse include in the care plan for a client who has moderate rheumatoid arthritis?

Select all that apply.

☐ **1.** Massaging inflamed joints

☐ **2.** Avoiding range-of-motion exercises

☐ **3.** Applying splints to inflamed joints

☐ **4.** Using assistive devices at all times

☐ **5.** Selecting clothing that has Velcro fasteners

☐ **6.** Applying moist heat to joints

Answer: 3, 5, 6

Rationale: Supportive, nonpharmacologic measures for the client with rheumatoid arthritis include applying splints to rest inflamed joints, using Velcro fasteners on clothes to aid in dressing, and applying moist heat to joints to relax muscles and relieve pain. Inflamed joints should never be massaged because doing so can aggravate inflammation. A physical therapy program including range-of-motion exercises and carefully individualized therapeutic exercises prevents loss of joint function. Assistive devices should only be used when marked loss of range of motion occurs.

Nursing process step: Planning

Client needs category: Physiological integrity

Client needs subcategory: Basic care and comfort

Cognitive level: Application

---

5. A nurse is assessing a client with a suspected Epstein-Barr viral infection. Identify the quadrant of the abdomen where the nurse is best able to palpate the spleen.

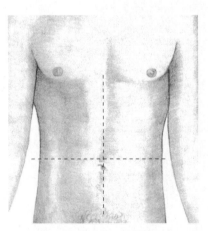

Answer:

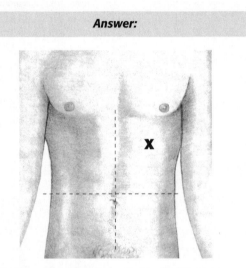

Rationale: The spleen is located in the left upper quadrant of the abdomen. It's posterior and slightly inferior to the stomach. The nurse should stop palpating immediately if she feels the spleen because compression can cause rupture.

Nursing process step: Assessment

Client needs category: Physiological integrity

Client needs subcategory: Physiological adaptation

Cognitive level: Application

6. A client has a viral infection and swollen lymph nodes. Identify the area where the nurse should place her hand to palpate the submandibular lymph nodes?

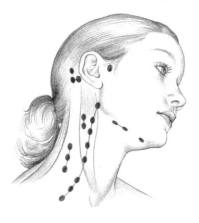

Answer:

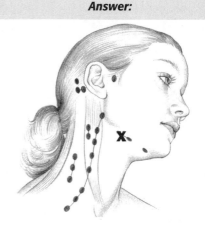

Rationale: The submandibular lymph nodes are found halfway between the angle and tip of the mandible.

Nursing process step: Assessment

Client needs category: Physiological integrity

Client needs subcategory: Physiological adaptation

Cognitive level: Application

Endocrine and metabolic disorders

1. A client is being discharged after having a thyroidectomy. Which of the following discharge instructions would be appropriate for this client?

Select all that apply.

☐ **1.** Report signs and symptoms of hypoglycemia.

☐ **2.** Take thyroid replacement medication as ordered.

☐ **3.** Watch for changes in body functioning, such as lethargy, restlessness, sensitivity to cold, and dry skin, and report these changes to the physician.

☐ **4.** Avoid all over-the-counter (OTC) medications.

☐ **5.** Carry injectable dexamethasone at all times.

Answer: 2, 3

Rationale: After removal of the thyroid gland, the client needs to take thyroid replacement medication. The client also needs to report such changes as lethargy, restlessness, cold sensitivity, and dry skin, which may indicate the need for a higher dosage of medication. The thyroid gland doesn't regulate blood glucose level; therefore, signs and symptoms of hypoglycemia aren't relevant for this client. Injectable dexamethasone isn't needed for this client. Some OTC medications (such as non-aspirin products) are allowable.

Nursing process step: Implementation

Client needs category: Physiological integrity

Client needs subcategory: Physiological adaptation

Cognitive level: Application

---

2. A client is admitted with a diagnosis of diabetic ketoacidosis. An insulin drip is initiated with 50 units of insulin in 100 ml of normal saline solution administered via an infusion pump set at 10 ml/hour. The nurse determines that the client is receiving how many units of insulin each hour?

_____

Answer: 5

Rationale: To determine the number of insulin units the client is receiving per hour, the nurse must first determine the number of units in each milliliter of fluid (50 units ÷ 100 ml = 0.5 unit/ml). Next, she multiplies the units per milliliter by the rate of milliliters per hour (0.5 unit × 10 ml/hr = 5 units).

Nursing process step: Analysis

Client needs category: Physiological integrity

Client needs subcategory: Pharmacological and parenteral therapies

Cognitive level: Application

---

3. A client's glucose level is 365 mg/dl. His physician orders 10 units of regular insulin to be administered. The bottle of regular insulin is labeled 100 units/ml. How many milliliters of insulin should a nurse administer?

_____

Answer: 0.1

Rationale: To find the correct administration amount, use the cross product principle to set up the following equation:

$$\frac{X}{10\ units} = \frac{1\ ml}{100\ units}$$

Next, cross-multiply:

$$100X\ units = 10\ units \times 1\ ml.$$

Then divide both sides of the equation by 100 units to solve for X:

$$X = 0.1\ ml.$$

Nursing process step: Implementation

Client needs category: Physiological integrity

Client needs subcategory: Pharmacological and parenteral therapies

Cognitive level: Application

4. A nurse is performing an admission assessment on a client who has been diagnosed with diabetes insipidus. Which of the following findings should the nurse expect to note during the assessment?

Select all that apply.

☐ **1.** Extreme polyuria

☐ **2.** Excessive thirst

☐ **3.** Elevated systolic blood pressure

☐ **4.** Low urine specific gravity

☐ **5.** Bradycardia

☐ **6.** Elevated serum potassium level

Answer: 1, 2, 4

Rationale: Signs and symptoms of diabetes insipidus include an abrupt onset of extreme polyuria, excessive thirst, dry skin and mucous membranes, tachycardia, and hypotension. Diagnostic studies reveal low urine specific gravity and osmolarity and an elevated serum sodium level. The serum potassium level is likely to be decreased, not increased.

Nursing process step: Assessment

Client needs category: Physiological integrity

Client needs subcategory: Physiological adaptation

Cognitive level: Comprehension

---

5. A client is being treated for hypothyroidism. Which of the following findings indicate that thyroid replacement therapy has been inadequate?

Select all that apply.

☐ **1.** Prolonged QT interval on electrocardiogram

☐ **2.** Tachycardia

☐ **3.** Low body temperature

☐ **4.** Nervousness

☐ **5.** Bradycardia

☐ **6.** Dry mouth

Answer: 1, 3, 5

Rationale: In hypothyroidism, the body is in a hypometabolic state. Therefore, a prolonged QT interval with bradycardia and subnormal body temperature would indicate that replacement therapy was inadequate. Tachycardia, nervousness, and dry mouth are symptoms of an excessive level of thyroid hormone; these findings would indicate that the client has received an excessive dose of thyroid hormone.

Nursing process step: Analysis

Client needs category: Physiological integrity

Client needs subcategory: Reduction of risk potential

Cognitive level: Analysis

6. A 55-year-old diabetic client is admitted with hypoglycemia. Which information should the nurse include in her client teaching?

Select all that apply.

☐ **1.** Hypoglycemia can result from excessive alcohol consumption.

☐ **2.** Skipping meals can cause hypoglycemia.

☐ **3.** Symptoms of hypoglycemia include thirst and excessive urination.

☐ **4.** Strenuous activity may result in hypoglycemia.

☐ **5.** Symptoms of hypoglycemia include shakiness, confusion, and headache.

☐ **6.** Hypoglycemia is a relatively harmless condition.

Answer: 1, 2, 4, 5

Rationale: Alcohol consumption, missed meals, and strenuous activity may lead to hypoglycemia. Symptoms of hypoglycemia include shakiness, confusion, headache, sweating, and tingling sensations around the mouth. Thirst and excessive urination are symptoms of hyperglycemia. Hypoglycemia can become a life-threatening disorder involving seizures and death of brain cells; the client shouldn't be told that the condition is relatively harmless.

Nursing process step: Implementation

Client needs category: Physiological integrity

Client needs subcategory: Reduction of risk potential

Cognitive level: Application

---

7. A nurse is caring for a client with a low calcium level. Prioritize the regulation of parathyroid hormone (PTH) release in relationship to low calcium levels.

| **1.** A high serum calcium level and inhibited PTH secretion |
| **2.** A low serum calcium level |
| **3.** Resorption of calcium |
| **4.** PTH release by the parathyroid gland |

| |
| |
| |
| |

Answer:

| **2.** A low serum calcium level |
| **4.** PTH release by the parathyroid gland |
| **3.** Resorption of calcium |
| **1.** A high serum calcium level and inhibited PTH secretion |

Rationale: Simple feedback occurs when the level of one substance regulates the secretion of hormones. A low calcium level stimulates the parathyroid gland to release PTH, which promotes resorption of calcium, resulting in normalized calcium levels. When calcium levels are elevated, PTH secretion is inhibited.

Nursing process step: Analysis

Client needs category: Physiological integrity

Client needs subcategory: Physiological adaptation

Cognitive level: Analysis

8. A client with Addison's disease is scheduled for discharge after being hospitalized for an adrenal crisis. Which statements by the client would indicate that client teaching has been effective?

Select all that apply.

☐ **1.** "I have to take my steroids for 10 days."

☐ **2.** "I need to weigh myself daily to be sure I don't eat too many calories."

☐ **3.** "I need to call my doctor to discuss my steroid needs before I have dental work."

☐ **4.** "I will call the doctor if I suddenly feel very weak or dizzy."

☐ **5.** "If I feel like I have the flu, I'll carry on as usual because this is an expected response."

☐ **6.** "I need to obtain and wear a Medic Alert bracelet."

Rationale: Dental work can be a cause of physical stress; therefore, the client's physician needs to be informed about the dental work so he can adjust the dosage of steroids if necessary. Fatigue, weakness, and dizziness are symptoms of inadequate steroid therapy; the physician should be notified if these symptoms occur. A Medic Alert bracelet allows health care providers to access the client's history of Addison's disease if the client is unable to communicate this information. A client with Addison's disease doesn't produce enough steroids, so routine administration of steroids is a lifetime treatment. Daily weight should be monitored to monitor changes in fluid balance, not calorie intake. Influenza is an added physical stressor that may require an increased dosage of steroids. The client should notify the physician, not "carry on as usual."

Nursing process step: Evaluation

Client needs category: Physiological integrity

Client needs subcategory: Reduction of risk potential

Cognitive level: Analysis

---

9. A client comes to the clinic because she has experienced a weight loss of 20 lb over the last month, even though her appetite has been "ravenous" and she hasn't changed her activity level. She's diagnosed with Graves' disease. For which other signs and symptoms of Graves' disease should the nurse assess the client?

Select all that apply.

☐ **1.** Rapid, bounding pulse

☐ **2.** Bradycardia

☐ **3.** Heat intolerance

☐ **4.** Mild tremors

☐ **5.** Nervousness

☐ **6.** Constipation

Rationale: Graves' disease, or hyperthyroidism, is a hypermetabolic state that's associated with a rapid, bounding pulse; heat intolerance; tremors; and nervousness. Bradycardia and constipation are signs and symptoms of hypothyroidism.

Nursing process step: Analysis

Client needs category: Health promotion and maintenance

Client needs subcategory: None

Cognitive level: Analysis

10. A client who suffered a brain injury after falling off a ladder has recently developed syndrome of inappropriate antidiuretic hormone (SIADH). Which findings indicate that the treatment he's receiving for SIADH is effective?

Select all that apply.

☐ **1.** Decrease in body weight

☐ **2.** Rise in blood pressure and drop in heart rate

☐ **3.** Absence of wheezing

☐ **4.** Increase in urine output

☐ **5.** Decrease in urine osmolarity

---

11. A nurse is about to administer a client's morning dose of insulin. The client's order is for 5 units of regular insulin and 10 units of NPH insulin given as a basal dose. He also is to receive an amount prescribed from his medium dose sliding scale (shown below) based on his morning blood glucose level. The nurse performs a bedside blood glucose measurement and the result is 264 mg/dl. How many total units of insulin should the nurse administer to the client?

Plasma glucose (mg/dl)	Low dose (regular insulin)	Medium dose (regular insulin)	High dose (regular insulin)	Very high dose (regular insulin)
< 70	←	Call physician		→
71-140	0 units	0 units	0 units	0 units
141-180	1 unit	2 units	4 units	10 units
181-240	2 units	4 units	8 units	15 units
241-300	4 units	6 units	12 units	20 units
301-400	6 units	9 units	16 units	25 units
> 400	8 units	12 units	20 units	30 units
	←	and call physician		→

Answer: 1, 4, 5

Rationale: SIADH is an abnormality involving an excessive release of antidiuretic hormone. The predominant feature is water retention with oliguria, edema, and weight gain. Successful treatment should result in a reduction in weight, increased urine output, and a decrease in urine osmolarity (concentration). Wheezes are not found in SIADH. Blood pressure would remain the same or decrease after treatment.

Nursing process step: Evaluation

Client needs category: Physiological integrity

Client needs subcategory: Physiological adaptation

Cognitive level: Analysis

Answer: 21

Rationale: The basal dose for this client is 5 units of regular insulin and 10 units of NPH insulin. The medium dose sliding scale indicates that glucose reading of 264 mg/dl should receive an additional 6 units of regular insulin, totalling 21 units (5 units + 10 units + 6 units = 21 units).

Nursing process step: Implementation

Client needs category: Physiological integrity

Client needs subcategory: Pharmacological and parenteral therapies

Cognitive level: Application

12. A client arrives in the clinic with a possible parathyroid hormone (PTH) deficiency. Diagnosis of this condition includes the analysis of serum electrolytes. Which of the following electrolytes would the nurse expect to be abnormal?

Select all that apply.

☐ **1.** Sodium

☐ **2.** Potassium

☐ **3.** Calcium

☐ **4.** Chloride

☐ **5.** Glucose

☐ **6.** Phosphorus

Answer: 3, 6

Rationale: A client with a PTH deficiency has abnormal calcium and phosphorus values because PTH regulates these two electrolytes. Sodium, chloride, potassium, and glucose aren't affected by a PTH deficiency.

Nursing process step: Evaluation

Client needs category: Health promotion and maintenance

Client needs subcategory: None

Cognitive level: Analysis

Musculoskeletal disorders

1. A client is diagnosed with osteoporosis. Which statements should the nurse include when teaching the client about the disease?

Select all that apply.

☐ **1.** It's common in females after menopause.

☐ **2.** It's a degenerative disease characterized by a decrease in bone density.

☐ **3.** It's a congenital disease caused by poor dietary intake of milk products.

☐ **4.** It can cause pain and injury.

☐ **5.** Passive range-of-motion exercises can promote bone growth.

☐ **6.** Weight-bearing exercise should be avoided.

Answer: 1, 2, 4

Rationale: Osteoporosis is a degenerative metabolic bone disorder in which the rate of bone resorption accelerates and the rate of bone formation decelerates, thus decreasing bone density. Postmenopausal women are at increased risk for this disorder because of their loss of estrogen. The decrease in bone density can cause pain and injury. Osteoporosis isn't a congenital disorder; however, low calcium intake does contribute to it. Passive range-of-motion exercises may be performed but they won't promote bone growth. The client should be encouraged to participate in weight-bearing exercise because it promotes bone growth.

Nursing process step: Implementation

Client needs category: Physiological integrity

Client needs subcategory: Physiological adaptation

Cognitive level: Application

2. A client is preparing for discharge after undergoing an above-the-knee amputation. Which of the following instructions should the nurse include in the teaching plan for this client?

Select all that apply.

☐ **1.** Massage the residual limb in a motion away from the suture line.

☐ **2.** Avoid using heat application to ease pain.

☐ **3.** Immediately report twitching, spasms, or phantom limb pain.

☐ **4.** Avoid exposing the skin around the residual limb to excessive perspiration.

☐ **5.** Be sure to perform the prescribed exercises.

☐ **6.** Rub the residual limb with a dry washcloth for 4 minutes three times daily if the limb is sensitive to touch.

Answer: 4, 5, 6

Rationale: The nurse should advise the client that perspiration on the residual limb may cause irritation. The client should exercise as instructed to minimize complications. In addition, rubbing the limb as described with a dry washcloth helps desensitize the skin. The nurse should instruct the client to massage the residual limb toward the suture line — not away from it — to mobilize the scar and prevent its adherence to bone. Twitching, spasms, or phantom limb pain are normal reactions to an amputation and don't need to be reported. The nurse should inform the client that these symptoms might be eased by heat, massage, or gentle pressure.

Nursing process step: Planning

Client needs category: Physiological integrity

Client needs subcategory: Reduction of risk potential

Cognitive level: Application

---

3. A client complains of an acute exacerbation of rheumatoid arthritis. The nurse plans care based on which of the following facts about rheumatoid arthritis?

Select all that apply.

☐ **1.** Onset is acute and usually occurs between ages 25 and 40.

☐ **2.** The client experiences stiff, swollen joints bilaterally.

☐ **3.** The client may not exercise once the disease is diagnosed.

☐ **4.** Erythrocyte sedimentation rate (ESR) is elevated and X-rays show erosions and decalcification of involved joints.

☐ **5.** Inflamed cartilage triggers complement activation, which stimulates the release of additional inflammatory mediators.

☐ **6.** The first-line treatment is gold salts and methotrexate.

Answer: 2, 4, 5

Rationale: Clients with rheumatoid arthritis experience stiff, swollen joints due to a severe inflammatory reaction. Elevated ESR and X-ray evidence of bony destruction are indicative of severe involvement. Rheumatoid arthritis starts insidiously, with fatigue, persistent low-grade fever, anorexia, and vague skeletal symptoms, usually between ages 35 and 50. Maintaining range of motion by a prescribed exercise program is essential, but clients must rest between activities. Salicylates and nonsteroidal anti-inflammatory drugs are considered the first-line treatment.

Nursing process step: Planning

Client needs category: Physiological Integrity

Client needs subcategory: Physiological adaptation

Cognitive level: Application

4. An elderly client fell and fractured the neck of his femur. Identify the area where the fracture occurred.

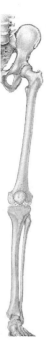

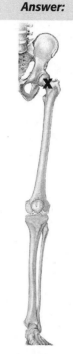

Rationale: The femur's neck connects the femur's round ball head to the shaft.

Nursing process step: Assessment

Client needs category: Physiological integrity

Client needs subcategory: Physiological adaptation

Cognitive level: Comprehension

---

5. A client is in the emergency department with a suspected fracture of the right hip. Which assessment findings of the right leg would the nurse expect?

Select all that apply.

☐ **1.** The right leg is longer than the left leg.

☐ **2.** The right leg is shorter than the left leg.

☐ **3.** The right leg is abducted.

☐ **4.** The right leg is adducted.

☐ **5.** The right leg is externally rotated.

☐ **6.** The right leg is internally rotated.

Answer: 2, 4, 5

Rationale: In a hip fracture, the affected leg is shorter, adducted, and externally rotated.

Nursing process step: Assessment

Client needs category: Physiological integrity

Client needs subcategory: Physiological adaptation

Cognitive level: Application

6. A client is scheduled for a laminectomy of the L1 and L2 vertebrae. Identify the area that's involved in the client's surgery.

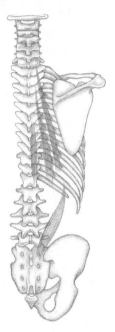

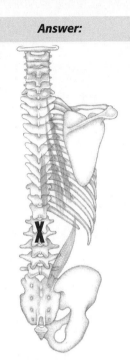

Rationale: In a laminectomy, one or more of the bony laminae that cover the vertebrae are removed. There are five lumbar vertebrae that are numbered from top to bottom. L5 is the closest to the sacrum. Count up from the sacrum to locate L1 and L2.

Nursing process step: Implementation

Client needs category: Physiological integrity

Client needs subcategory: Physiological adaptation

Cognitive level: Comprehension

---

7. A client is diagnosed with gout. Which foods should the nurse instruct the client to avoid?

Select all that apply.

☐ **1.** Green leafy vegetables

☐ **2.** Liver

☐ **3.** Cod

☐ **4.** Chocolate

☐ **5.** Sardines

☐ **6.** Eggs

Answer: 2, 3, 5

Rationale: Clients with gout should avoid foods that are high in purines, such as liver, cod, and sardines. They should also avoid anchovies, kidneys, sweetbreads, lentils, and alcoholic beverages — especially beer and wine. Green leafy vegetables, chocolate, and eggs aren't high in purines.

Nursing process step: Implementation

Client needs category: Physiological integrity

Client needs subcategory: Basic care and comfort

Cognitive level: Application

Neurosensory disorders

1. A nurse is preparing a female client with tonic-clonic seizure disorder for discharge. Which instructions should the nurse include about phenytoin (Dilantin)?

Select all that apply.

☐ **1.** Monitor for skin rash.

☐ **2.** Maintain adequate amounts of fluid and fiber in the diet.

☐ **3.** Perform good oral hygiene, including daily brushing and flossing.

☐ **4.** Receive necessary periodic blood work.

☐ **5.** Report to the physician any problems with walking or coordination, slurred speech, or nausea.

☐ **6.** Feel safe about taking this drug, even during pregnancy.

> *Answer: 1, 3, 4, 5*

Rationale: A rash may occur 10 to 14 days after starting phenytoin. If a rash appears, the client should notify the physician and discontinue the medication. Because phenytoin may cause gingival hyperplasia, the client must practice good oral hygiene and see a dentist regularly. Periodic blood work is necessary to monitor complete blood counts, platelet count, hepatic function, and drug levels. Signs and symptoms of phenytoin toxicity include problems with walking or coordination, slurred speech, and nausea. Other signs of toxicity include lethargy, diplopia, nystagmus, and disturbances in balance. These symptoms must be reported to the physician immediately. Although adequate amounts of fluid and fiber are part of a healthy diet, they aren't required for a client taking phenytoin. Phenytoin must be used cautiously during pregnancy because it poses an increased risk of birth defects; phenobarbital is a safer drug to take during pregnancy.

Nursing process step: Implementation

Client needs category: Physiological integrity

Client needs subcategory: Pharmacological and parenteral therapies

Cognitive level: Application

---

2. A nurse is assessing a 21-year-old client diagnosed with bacterial meningitis. Which of the following signs and symptoms of meningeal irritation is the nurse likely to observe?

Select all that apply.

☐ **1.** Generalized seizures

☐ **2.** Nuchal rigidity

☐ **3.** Positive Brudzinski's sign

☐ **4.** Positive Kernig's sign

☐ **5.** Babinski's reflex

☐ **6.** Photophobia

> *Answer: 2, 3, 4, 6*

Rationale: Signs of meningeal irritation include nuchal rigidity, positive Brudzinski's and Kernig's signs, and photophobia. Other signs of meningeal irritation are exaggerated and symmetrical deep tendon reflexes as well as opisthotonos (a spasm in which the back and extremities arch backward so that the body rests on the head and heals). Generalized seizures, which may accompany meningitis, are caused by irritation to the cerebral cortex, not the meninges. Babinski's reflex is a reflex action of the toes that reflects corticospinal tract disease in adults.

Nursing process step: Assessment

Client needs category: Physiological integrity

Client needs subcategory: Physiological adaptation

Cognitive level: Application

3. A nurse is preparing to administer phenytoin (Dilantin) to a client with a seizure disorder. The order is for phenytoin 5 mg/kg/day to be administered in divided doses. The client weighs 99 lb and the medication will be administered three times per day. How many milligrams of phenytoin should be administered in the first dose?

_____

Answer: 75

Rationale: First, convert the client's weight to kilograms:

$$1 \text{ kg} = 2.2 \text{ lb}$$

$$99 \text{ lb} \div 2.2 \text{ lb/kg} = 44 \text{ kg.}$$

Then calculate the total daily dosage:

$$44 \text{ kg} \times 5 \text{ mg/kg} = 220 \text{ mg/day.}$$

Finally, divide the total daily dosage into three parts:

$$220 \text{ mg} \div 3 \text{ doses} = 75 \text{ mg/dose.}$$

Nursing process step: Implementation

Client needs category: Physiological integrity

Client needs subcategory: Pharmacological and parenteral therapies

Cognitive level: Application

---

4. A nurse is assessing a client's extraocular eye movements as part of the neurologic examination. Which of the following cranial nerves is the nurse assessing?

Select all that apply.

☐ **1.** Optic (II)

☐ **2.** Oculomotor (III)

☐ **3.** Trochlear (IV)

☐ **4.** Trigeminal (V)

☐ **5.** Abducens (VI)

☐ **6.** Acoustic (VIII)

Answer: 2, 3, 5

Rationale: Assessing extraocular eye movements helps evaluate the function of cranial nerves III (oculomotor), IV (trochlear), and VI (abducens). The oculomotor nerve originates in the brainstem and controls the movement of the eyeball up, down, and inward; raises the eyelid; and constricts the pupil. The trochlear nerve rotates the eyeball downward and outward. The abducens nerve originates in the pons and rotates the eyeball laterally. Assessing the client's vision helps evaluate cranial nerve II (optic). Cranial nerve V (trigeminal), has three branches: assessing the corneal reflex helps the nurse evaluate the ophthalmic branch functions; assessing sensation to the cheek, upper jaw, teeth, lips, hard palate, maxillary sinus, and part of the nasal mucosa helps evaluate the maxillary branch functions; and assessing sensation to the lower lip, chin, ear, mucous membrane, lower teeth, and tongue helps evaluate the mandibular branch functions. Assessing hearing and balance helps evaluate the cochlear and vestibular branches of cranial nerve VIII (acoustic).

Nursing process step: Assessment

Client needs category: Physiological integrity

Client needs subcategory: Physiological adaptation

Cognitive level: Analysis

5. A nurse is assessing the level of consciousness of a client who suffered a head injury. Using the Glasgow Coma Scale, she determines that the client's score is 15. Which of the following responses did the nurse assess in this client?

Select all that apply.

☐ **1.** Spontaneous eye opening

☐ **2.** Tachypnea, bradycardia, and hypotension

☐ **3.** Unequal pupil size

☐ **4.** Orientation to person, place, and time

☐ **5.** Pain localized

☐ **6.** Incomprehensible sounds

Answer: 1, 4

Rationale: To achieve a perfect 15 score on the Glasgow Coma Scale, the client would have to open his eyes spontaneously (4), obey verbal commands (6), and be oriented to person, place, and time (5). Vital signs and pupil size aren't assessed with the Glasgow Coma Scale. The ability to localize pain earns a motor response score of 5, not the top score of 6. Making incomprehensible sounds earns a verbal response score of 2, not a 5.

Nursing process step: Analysis

Client needs category: Physiological integrity

Client needs subcategory: Physiological adaptation

Cognitive level: Analysis

---

6. A nurse is assessing a client using the Glasgow Coma Scale (shown below). The client complains of pain in his abdominal area; is confused about person, place, and time; and anxiously watches the nurse as she performs the assessment. Using the scale provided, what score should this client receive?

Glasgow Coma Scale

Test	Client's reaction	Score
Eye opening response	Opens spontaneously	4
	Opens to verbal command	3
	Opens to pain	2
	No response	1
Best motor response	Obeys verbal command	6
	Localizes painful stimuli	5
	Flexion-withdrawal	4
	Flexion-abnormal (decorticate rigidity)	3
	Extension (decerebrate rigidity)	2
	No response	1
Best verbal response	Oriented and converses	5
	Disoriented and converses	4
	Inappropriate words	3
	Incomprehensible sounds	2
	No response	1

☐ **1.** 9

☐ **2.** 11

☐ **3.** 13

☐ **4.** 15

Answer: 3

Rationale: The Glasgow Coma Scale assesses level of consciousness by testing and scoring the client's best eye opening, motor, and verbal responses. The highest score is 15. In this case, the client spontaneously keeps his eyes open as he watches the actions of the nurse (eye opening score of 4), can express and localize the area of his pain (motor response score of 5), and is disoriented about person, place, and time (verbal response score of 4) for a total score of 13.

Nursing process step: Assessment

Client needs category: Physiological integrity

Client needs subcategory: Physiological adaptation

Cognitive level: Analysis

7. A nurse is caring for a client with a T5 complete spinal cord injury. Upon assessment, the nurse notes flushed skin, diaphoresis above T5, and blood pressure of 162/96 mm Hg. The client reports a severe, pounding headache. Which of the following nursing interventions would be appropriate for this client?

Select all that apply.

☐ **1.** Elevate the head of the bed to 90 degrees.

☐ **2.** Loosen constrictive clothing.

☐ **3.** Use a fan to reduce diaphoresis.

☐ **4.** Assess for bladder distention and bowel impaction.

☐ **5.** Administer antihypertensive medication.

☐ **6.** Place the client in a supine position with legs elevated.

Answer: 1, 2, 4, 5

Rationale: The client is exhibiting signs and symptoms of autonomic dysreflexia, a potentially life-threatening emergency caused by an uninhibited response from the sympathetic nervous system resulting from a lack of control over the autonomic nervous system. The nurse should immediately elevate the head of the bed to 90 degrees and place the legs in a dependent position to decrease venous return to the heart and increase venous return from the brain. Because tactile stimuli can trigger autonomic dysreflexia, any constrictive clothing should be loosened. The nurse should also assess for distended bladder and bowel impaction — which may trigger autonomic dysreflexia — and correct any problems. Elevated blood pressure is the most life-threatening complication of autonomic dysreflexia because it can cause stroke, myocardial infarction, or seizure activity. If removing the triggering event doesn't reduce the client's blood pressure, I.V. antihypertensives should be administered. A fan shouldn't be used because a cold draft may trigger autonomic dysreflexia.

Nursing process step: Implementation

Client needs category: Physiological integrity

Client needs subcategory: Reduction of risk potential

Cognitive level: Application

8. A client has a cerebral aneurysm. The physician orders hydralazine (Apresoline) 15 mg I.V. every 4 hours as needed to keep the systolic blood pressure less than 140 mm Hg. The label on the hydralazine vial reads "hydralazine 20 mg/ml." To administer the correct dose, how many milliliters of medication should the nurse draw up in the syringe?

Answer: 0.75

Rationale: The following formula is used to calculate drug dosages:

Dose on hand/Quantity on hand = Dose desired/X

20 mg/ml = 15 mg/X = 0.75 ml.

Nursing process step: Implementation

Client needs category: Physiological integrity

Client needs subcategory: Pharmacological and parenteral therapies

Cognitive level: Application

9. A nurse is preparing to teach students in a health class about hearing pathways. Prioritize the steps she'll describe that explain how sound wave transmission allows an individual to hear.

1.	Interpretation of sound by the cerebral cortex

2.	Transmission of vibrations through the air and bone

3.	Stimulation of nerve impulses in the inner ear

4.	Transmission of vibrations to the auditory area of the cerebral cortex

Answer:

2.	Transmission of vibrations through the air and bone

3.	Stimulation of nerve impulses in the inner ear

4.	Transmission of vibrations to the auditory area of the cerebral cortex

1.	Interpretation of sound by the cerebral cortex

Rationale: Vibrations transmitted through air and bone stimulate nerve impulses in the inner ear. The cochlear branch of the acoustic nerve transmits these vibrations to the auditory area of the cerebral cortex. The cerebral cortex then interprets the sound.

Nursing process step: Implementation

Client needs category: Health promotion and maintenance

Client needs subcategory: None

Cognitive level: Application

---

10. A community nurse is leading a discussion with clients in a support group on the progressive nature of multiple sclerosis (MS). Arrange the degenerative changes shown below in the order in which they occur.

1.	Degeneration of axons

2.	Demyelination throughout the central nervous system

3.	Periodic and unpredictable exacerbations and remissions

4.	Plaque formation that interrupts nerve impulses

Answer:

2.	Demyelination throughout the central nervous system

1.	Degeneration of axons

4.	Plaque formation that interrupts nerve impulses

3.	Periodic and unpredictable exacerbations and remissions

Rationale: MS produces patches of demyelination throughout the central nervous system, resulting in myelin loss from the axis cylinders and degeneration of the axons. Plaques form in the involved area and become sclerosed, interrupting the flow of nerve impulses and resulting in a variety of symptoms. Periodic and unpredictable exacerbations and remissions occur. The prognosis varies.

Nursing process step: Implementation

Client needs category: Physiological integrity

Client needs subcategory: Physiological adaptation

Cognitive level: Application

11. A nurse is monitoring a client's intracranial pressure (ICP) after a traumatic head injury. Based on the documentation below, how should the nurse interpret this client's ICP reading?

	0800	0805	0810	0815
ICP	20	18	18	16

☐ **1.** ICP is elevated.

☐ **2.** ICP is decreased.

☐ **3.** ICP is within normal limits.

☐ **4.** ICP was elevated but returned to normal.

Rationale: A normal ICP is between 0 and 15 mm Hg. The documentation at left shows pressures greater than 15 mm Hg.

Nursing process step: Assessment

Client needs category: Physiological integrity

Client needs subcategory: Reduction of risk potential

Cognitive level: Analysis

---

12. A client is experiencing problems with balance as well as fine and gross motor function. Which area of the brain is malfunctioning?

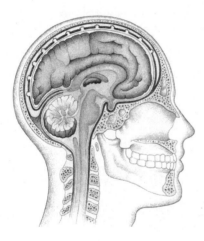

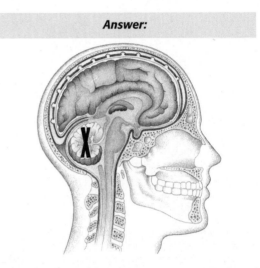

Rationale: The cerebellum is the portion of the brain that controls balance and fine and gross motor function.

Nursing process step: Assessment

Client needs category: Physiological integrity

Client needs subcategory: Reduction of risk potential

Cognitive level: Comprehension

13. A nurse is performing a neurologic assessment on a client during a routine physical examination. To assess Babinski's reflex, indicate the point where the nurse would place the tongue blade to begin stroking the foot.

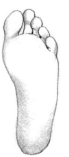

Answer:

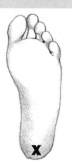

Rationale: To test for Babinski's reflex, use a tongue blade to slowly stroke the side of the sole of the foot. Start at the heel and move towards the great toe. The normal response in an adult is plantar flexion of the toes. Upward movement of the great toe and fanning of the little toes — Babinski's reflex — is abnormal.

Nursing process step: Assessment

Client needs category: Health promotion and maintenance

Client needs subcategory: None

Cognitive level: Comprehension

Respiratory disorders

1. A nurse is caring for a client with pneumonia who was prescribed ceftriaxone (Rocephin) oral suspension 600 mg once daily. The medication label indicates that the strength is 125 mg/5 ml. How many milliliters of medication should the nurse pour to administer the correct dose?

Answer: 24

Rationale: The following formula is used to calculate drug dosages:

Dose on hand/Quantity on hand = Dose desired/X.

Plug in the values for this equation:

125 mg/5 ml = 600 mg/X.

X = 24 ml.

Nursing process step: Planning

Client needs category: Physiological integrity

Client needs subcategory: Pharmacological and parenteral therapies

Cognitive level: Application

2. A nurse is caring for a client who has a chest tube connected to a three-chamber drainage system without suction. On the illustration below, identify the chamber that collects drainage from the client.

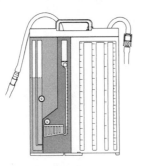

Answer:

Answer:

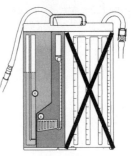

Rationale: The drainage system is on the right. It has three calibrated chambers that show the amount of drainage collected. When the first chamber fills, drainage empties into the second; when the second chamber fills, drainage flows into the third. The water seal chamber is located in the center. The suction control chamber is on the left.

Nursing process step: Implementation

Client needs category: Physiological integrity

Client needs subcategory: Reduction of risk potential

Cognitive level: Comprehension

---

3. A client comes to the emergency department with status asthmaticus. Based on the documentation note below, the nurse suspects that the client has what abnormality?

1/11/06	Pt. wheezing. RR 44, BP 140/90, P 104,
1830	T 98.4° F. ABG results show pH 7.52, Paco₂
	30 mm Hg, HCO₃⁻ 26 mEq/L, and PO₂
	77 mm Hg. ———————— C. Wynn, RN

☐ **1.** Respiratory acidosis

☐ **2.** Respiratory alkalosis

☐ **3.** Metabolic acidosis

☐ **4.** Metabolic alkalosis

Answer: 2

Rationale: Respiratory alkalosis results from alveolar hyperventilation. It's marked by an increase in pH to more than 7.45 and a concurrent decrease in partial pressure of arterial carbon dioxide ($Paco_2$) to less than 35 mm Hg. Metabolic alkalosis shows the same increase in pH but also an increased bicarbonate level and normal $Paco_2$ (may be elevated also if compensatory mechanisms are working). Acidosis of any type means a low pH (below 7.35). Respiratory acidosis shows an elevated $Paco_2$ and a normal to high bicarbonate level. Metabolic acidosis is characterized by a decreased bicarbonate level and a normal to low $Paco_2$.

Nursing process step: Analysis

Client needs category: Physiological integrity

Client needs subcategory: Physiological adaptation

Cognitive level: Analysis

4. A nurse is preparing a staff education program about pulmonary circulation. Place the options below into the order that matches the path of pulmonary circulation.

| 1. Pulmonary vein |
| 2. Right ventricle |
| 3. Pulmonary artery |
| 4. Arterioles |
| 5. Alveoli |
| 6. Left atrium |

| 2. Right ventricle |
| 3. Pulmonary artery |
| 4. Arterioles |
| 5. Alveoli |
| 1. Pulmonary vein |
| 6. Left atrium |

Rationale: The pulmonary artery takes deoxygenated blood from the right ventricle to the lungs via the arterioles and alveoli. The pulmonary vein carries oxygenated blood back to the left atrium for circulation throughout the body.

Nursing process step: Analysis

Client needs category: Physiological integrity

Client needs subcategory: Physiological adaptation

Cognitive level: Comprehension

---

5. A client with a suspected pulmonary embolus is brought to the emergency department. She complains of shortness of breath and chest pain. For which other signs and symptoms would the nurse assess the client?

Select all that apply.

☐ **1.** Low-grade fever

☐ **2.** Thick green sputum

☐ **3.** Bradycardia

☐ **4.** Frothy sputum

☐ **5.** Tachycardia

☐ **6.** Blood-tinged sputum

Answer: 1, 5, 6

Rationale: In addition to pleuritic chest pain and dyspnea, a client with a pulmonary embolus may present with a low-grade fever, tachycardia, and blood-tinged sputum. Thick green sputum would indicate infection, and frothy sputum would indicate pulmonary edema. A client with a pulmonary embolus is tachycardic (to compensate for decreased oxygen supply), not bradycardic.

Nursing process step: Assessment

Client needs category: Physiological integrity

Client needs subcategory: Physiological adaptation

Cognitive level: Application

6. A client with chronic obstructive pulmonary disease (COPD) is being evaluated for a lung transplant. Which signs and symptoms should the nurse expect to find in the initial physical assessment?

Select all that apply.

☐ **1.** Decreased respiratory rate

☐ **2.** Dyspnea on exertion

☐ **3.** Barrel chest

☐ **4.** Shortened expiratory phase

☐ **5.** Clubbed fingers and toes

☐ **6.** Fever

Answer: 2, 3, 5

Rationale: Typical findings for clients with COPD include dyspnea on exertion, a barrel chest, and clubbed fingers and toes. Clients with COPD are usually tachypneic with a prolonged expiratory phase. Fever is not associated with COPD, unless an infection is also present.

Nursing process step: Assessment

Client needs category: Physiological integrity

Client needs subcategory: Physiological adaptation

Cognitive level: Application

---

7. A client with a wound infection develops septic shock. An arterial blood gas analysis reveals pH of 7.25, partial pressure of arterial carbon dioxide ($Paco_2$) of 43 mm Hg, partial pressure of arterial oxygen (Pao_2) of 70 mm Hg, and bicarbonate (HCO_3^-) of 18 mEq/L. According to the following oxyhemoglobin dissociation curve, which statement is correct?

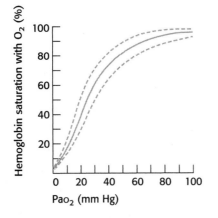

Pao₂ (mm Hg)

☐ **1.** The client's profile reflects alkalosis.

☐ **2.** The client's hemoglobin saturation is close to 100%.

☐ **3.** The client's oxyhemoglobin curve is shifted to the left.

☐ **4.** The client's hemoglobin saturation is close to 85%.

Answer: 4

Rationale: The acidic condition of the blood shifts the oxyhemoglobin dissociation curve to the right. This enables oxygen molecules to unload more easily from the hemoglobin. According to the client's Pao_2 value of 70 mm Hg and pH value, his hemoglobin saturation is close to 85%.

Nursing process step: Analysis

Client needs category: Physiological integrity

Client needs subcategory: Physiological adaptation

Cognitive level: Analysis

8. A client with a traumatic injury who is in the intensive care unit develops a tension pneumothorax. The nurse is aware that which of the following signs and symptoms are associated with tension pneumothorax?

Select all that apply.

☐ **1.** Decreased cardiac output

☐ **2.** Flattened neck veins

☐ **3.** Tracheal deviation to the affected side

☐ **4.** Hypotension

☐ **5.** Tracheal deviation to the opposite side

☐ **6.** Bradypnea

Answer: 1, 4, 5

Rationale: Tension pneumothorax results when air in the pleural space is under higher pressure than air in the adjacent lung. The site of the rupture of the pleural space acts as a one-way valve, allowing the air to enter on inspiration but not escape on expiration. The air presses against the mediastinum, causing a tracheal shift to the opposite side and decreased venous return (reflected by decreased cardiac output and hypotension). Neck veins bulge with tension pneumothorax. This also leads to compensatory tachycardia and tachypnea.

Nursing process step: Assessment

Client needs category: Physiological integrity

Client needs subcategory: Physiological adaptation

Cognitive level: Application

---

9. A client with right-middle-lobe pneumonia is being cared for in the intensive care unit. In the anterior view of the lungs, below, identify the area where the nurse may expect to hear associated adventitious breath sounds such as crackles.

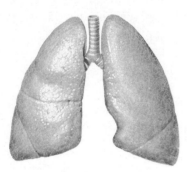

Answer:

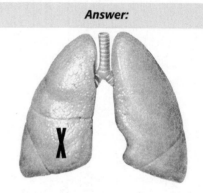

Rationale: The right lung is made up of three lobes: the right upper lobe, right middle lobe, and right lower lobe. The left lung is made up of only two lobes: the left upper lobe and the left lower lobe. When assessing the anterior chest, the right lung is on the examiner's left.

Nursing process step: Assessment

Client needs category: Health promotion and maintenance

Client needs subcategory: None

Cognitive level: Analysis

10. A client is prescribed continuous positive airway pressure (CPAP) therapy for sleep apnea. Identify the location where the mechanism maintaining the positive end-expiratory pressure is located.

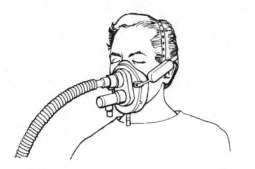

Answer:

Rationale: CPAP ventilation maintains positive pressure in the airways throughout the respiratory cycle. The inlet valve attaches the oxygen tubing to the face mask, and the positive end-expiratory pressure valve maintains the pressure. CPAP can be used with or without a ventilator in intubated and nonintubated clients and can be administered just nasally for a less constrictive feeling. In addition to sleep apnea, CPAP is used to treat respiratory distress syndrome, pulmonary edema, pulmonary emboli, bronchiolitis, pneumonitis, viral pneumonia, and postoperative atelectasis.

Nursing process step: Planning

Client needs category: Physiological integrity

Client needs subcategory: Physiological adaptation

Cognitive level: Application

---

11. A client with primary pulmonary hypertension is being evaluated for a heart-lung transplant. The nurse would expect the client to be receiving which treatments?

Select all that apply.

☐ **1.** Oxygen

☐ **2.** Aminoglycosides

☐ **3.** Diuretics

☐ **4.** Vasodilators

☐ **5.** Antihistamines

☐ **6.** Sulfonamides

Answer: 1, 3, 4

Rationale: Oxygen, diuretics, and vasodilators are among the common therapies used to treat pulmonary hypertension. Others include fluid restriction, digoxin, calcium channel blockers, beta-adrenergic blockers, and bronchodilators. Aminoglycosides and sulfonamides are antibiotics used to treat infections. Antihistamines are indicated to treat allergies, pruritus, vertigo, nausea, and vomiting; to promote sedation; and to suppress cough.

Nursing process step: Implementation

Client needs category: Physiological integrity

Client needs subcategory: Pharmacological and parenteral therapies

Cognitive level: Application

12. A nurse is performing a respiratory assessment on a client with right-lower-lobe atelectasis. Identify the area where she may hear the fine crackles associated with this condition.

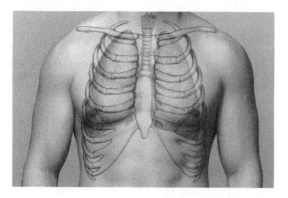

Answer:

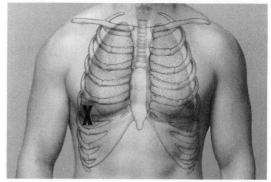

Rationale: To auscultate the right lower lobe from the anterior chest, the nurse should place the stethoscope between the fifth and sixth intercostal spaces to the left of the anterior axillary line.

Nursing process step: Assessment

Client needs category: Physiological integrity

Client needs subcategory: Reduction of risk potential

Cognitive level: Application

Genitourinary disorders

1. A 176-lb client with minimal urine output has been prescribed dopamine at 5 mcg/kg/minute. The premixed bag of dopamine contains 800 mg in 500 ml dextrose 5% in water. How many milliliters of the solution containing dopamine should the nurse administer each hour?

Answer: 15

Rationale: Factor analysis is the easiest way to solve this problem. Identify the information you have, and then use conversion factors to obtain the information you need.

$$\frac{176 \text{ lb}}{1} \times \frac{1 \text{ kg}}{2.2 \text{ lb}} \times \frac{5 \text{ mcg}}{1 \text{ kg/min}} \times \frac{1 \text{ mg}}{1000 \text{ mcg}} \times \frac{500 \text{ ml}}{800 \text{ mg}} \times \frac{60 \text{ min}}{1 \text{ hr}}$$

$$\frac{26,400,000 \text{ ml}}{1,760,000 \text{ hr}} = 15 \text{ ml/hr}$$

Nursing process step: Implementation

Client needs category: Physiological integrity

Client needs subcategory: Pharmacological and parenteral therapies

Cognitive level: Application

2. A client with marked oliguria is ordered a test dose of 0.2 g/kg of 15% mannitol solution I.V. over 5 minutes. The patient weighs 132 lb. How many grams should the nurse administer?

_____

Answer: 12

Rationale: First, the nurse should convert the client's weight from grams to kilograms:

$$132 \text{ lb} \div 2.2 \text{ kg/lb} = 60 \text{ kg}.$$

Then, to calculate the number of grams to administer, the nurse should multiply the ordered number of grams by the patient's weight in kilograms:

$$0.2 \text{ g/kg} \times 60 \text{ kg} = 12 \text{ g}.$$

Nursing process step: Implementation

Client needs category: Physiological integrity

Client needs subcategory: Pharmacological and parenteral therapies

Cognitive level: Analysis

---

3. A nurse is providing health teaching to a client with benign prostatic hyperplasia. Identify the area where the nurse would indicate that the prostate gland is located.

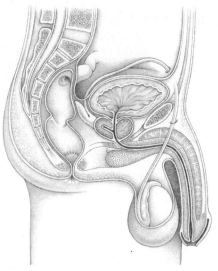

Answer:

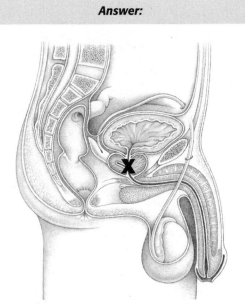

Rationale: The walnut-sized prostate gland lies beneath the bladder and surrounds the urethra.

Nursing process step: Assessment

Client needs category: Physiological integrity

Client needs subcategory: Physiological adaptation

Cognitive level: Application

4. After a retropubic prostatectomy, a client needs continuous bladder irrigation. The client has an I.V. of dextrose in 5% water infusing at 40 ml/hr and a triple-lumen urinary catheter with normal saline solution infusing at 200 ml/hr. The nurse empties the urinary catheter drainage bag three times during an 8-hour period for a total of 2,780 ml. How many milliliters does the nurse calculate as urine?

_____

Rationale: During 8 hours, 1,600 ml of bladder irrigant has been infused (200 ml × 8 hr = 1,600 ml/8 hr). The nurse should subtract this amount from the total volume in the drainage bag to determine urine output (2,780 ml − 1,600 ml = 1,180 ml).

Nursing process step: Implementation

Client needs category: Physiological integrity

Client needs subcategory: Basic care and comfort

Cognitive level: Analysis

---

5. A nurse is caring for a client with chronic renal failure. The laboratory results indicate hypocalcemia and hyperphosphatemia. When assessing the client, the nurse should be alert for which of the following?

Select all that apply.

☐ **1.** Trousseau's sign

☐ **2.** Cardiac arrhythmias

☐ **3.** Constipation

☐ **4.** Decreased clotting time

☐ **5.** Drowsiness and lethargy

☐ **6.** Fractures

Answer: 1, 2, 6

Rationale: Hypocalcemia is a calcium deficit that causes nerve fiber irritability and repetitive muscle spasms. Signs and symptoms of hypocalcemia include Trousseau's sign, cardiac arrhythmias, diarrhea, increased clotting times, anxiety, and irritability. The calcium-phosphorus imbalance leads to brittle bones and pathologic fractures. Drowsiness and lethargy are not typically associated with hypercalcemia.

Nursing process step: Assessment

Client needs category: Physiological integrity

Client needs subcategory: Reduction of risk potential

Cognitive level: Application

6. A nurse is explaining menstruation to a class. Place the pathophysiologic steps of the menstrual cycle listed below in the correct order.

1.	The level of estrogen in the blood peaks.

2.	Peak endometrial thickening occurs.

3.	Increased estrogen and progesterone levels inhibit luteinizing hormone.

4.	The top layer of the endometrium breaks down and sloughs.

5.	A follicle matures and ovulation occurs.

6.	The endometrium begins thickening.

4.	The top layer of the endometrium breaks down and sloughs.

6.	The endometrium begins thickening.

1.	The level of estrogen in the blood peaks.

5.	A follicle matures and ovulation occurs.

2.	Peak endometrial thickening occurs.

3.	Increased estrogen and progesterone levels inhibit luteinizing hormone.

Rationale: The menstrual cycle begins with the first day of menstruation and progresses through the steps described above. Increased estrogen and progesterone inhibit-follicle stimulating hormone, which causes a feedback loop that then decreases estrogen and progesterone production. This causes the top layer of endometrium to break down and slough, restarting the cycle in a nonpregnant female.

Nursing process step: Planning

Client needs category: Health promotion and maintenance

Client needs subcategory: None

Cognitive level: Application

PART THREE

Maternal-infant nursing

Antepartum period

1. During her first prenatal visit, a client asks a nurse what physiological changes she can expect during pregnancy. The nurse begins the discussion with the presumptive changes of pregnancy. Put the following presumptive changes in ascending chronological order.

1. Frequent urination

2. Breast changes

3. Quickening

4. Linea nigra, melasma, and striae gravidarum

5. Uterine enlargement in which the uterus can be palpated over the symphysis pubis

Answer:

2. Breast changes

1. Frequent urination

5. Uterine enlargement in which the uterus can be palpated over the symphysis pubis

3. Quickening

4. Linea nigra, melasma, and striae gravidarum

Rationale: Presumptive changes are subjective and can be caused by other medical conditions. Breast changes occur approximately 2 weeks after implantation of the embryo; frequent urination, at 3 weeks; fatigue and uterine enlargement over the symphysis pubis, at 18 weeks; quickening, between 18 and 20 weeks; and linea nigra, melasma, and striae gravidarum, at 24 weeks.

Nursing process step: Implementation

Client needs category: Health promotion and maintenance

Client needs subcategory: None

Cognitive level: Application

---

2. A 30-year-old client comes to the office for a routine prenatal visit. After reading the chart entry below, the nurse should prepare the client for which of the following studies?

6/8/06	Pt. is 11 weeks pregnant; urine sample shows
1320	glycosuria. Pt. has a family history of
	diabetes. ———— Chrissy Franks, RN

☐ **1.** Triple screen

☐ **2.** Indirect Coombs test

☐ **3.** 1-hour glucose tolerance test

☐ **4.** Amniocentesis

Answer: 3

Rationale: A 1-hour glucose tolerance test is recommended to screen for gestational diabetes if the client is obese, has glycosuria or a family history of diabetes, or lost a fetus for unexplained reasons or gave birth to a large-for-gestational-age neonate. A triple screen tests for chromosomal abnormalities. The indirect Coombs test screens maternal blood for red blood cell antibodies. Amniocentesis is used to detect fetal abnormalities.

Nursing process step: Analysis

Client needs category: Physiological integrity

Client needs subcategory: Reduction of risk potential

Cognitive level: Application

3. A nurse is preparing to teach a client about fetal growth and development during the first 3 months of pregnancy. Help prepare the teaching materials by putting the following milestones in order by month (month 1, month 2, month 3, and months 4 to 9).

1. Teeth and bones begin to appear, the kidneys start to function and, at the end of the month, gender is distinguishable.

2. The embryo has a definite form; the head, trunk, and tiny buds for arms and legs develop; and the cardiovascular system begins to function.

3. Internal and external fetal growth continues at a rapid rate, and the fetus stores the fats and minerals it needs to live outside the womb.

4. The eyes, ears, nose, lips, tongue, and tooth buds develop; the umbilical cord has a definite form; and the external genitalia are present.

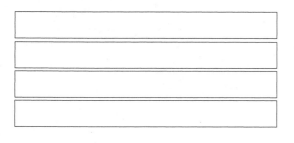

Answer:

2. The embryo has a definite form; the head, trunk, and tiny buds for arms and legs develop; and the cardiovascular system begins to function.

4. The eyes, ears, nose, lips, tongue, and tooth buds develop; the umbilical cord has a definite form; and the external genitalia are present.

1. Teeth and bones begin to appear, the kidneys start to function and, at the end of the month, gender is distinguishable.

3. Internal and external fetal growth continues at a rapid rate, and the fetus stores the fats and minerals it needs to live outside the womb.

Rationale: Significant growth and development take place during the first 3 months, in the order listed above. During the last 6 months, growth continues until the fetus is full-term.

Nursing process step: Planning

Client needs category: Health promotion and maintenance

Client needs subcategory: None

Cognitive level: Application

---

4. A woman who is 15 weeks pregnant comes to the clinic for amniocentesis. The nurse knows that this test can be used to identify which of the following characteristics or problems?

Select all that apply.

☐ **1.** Fetal lung maturity

☐ **2.** Gestational diabetes

☐ **3.** Chromosomal defects

☐ **4.** Neural tube defects

☐ **5.** Polyhydramnios

☐ **6.** Sex of the fetus

Answer: 3, 4, 6

Rationale: In early pregnancy, amniocentesis can be used to identify chromosomal and neural tube defects and determine the sex of the fetus. It can be used to evaluate fetal lung maturity during the last trimester of pregnancy. A blood test performed between 24 and 28 weeks' gestation is used to screen for gestational diabetes. Ultrasound is used to identify polyhydramnios; amniocentesis can be used to treat polyhydramnios by removing excess fluid.

Nursing process step: Planning

Client needs category: Physiological integrity

Client needs subcategory: Reduction of risk potential

Cognitive level: Application

5. A client who is 41 weeks pregnant is about to undergo a biophysical profile (BPP) to evaluate her fetus's well-being. A nurse knows that which of the following components are included in a BPP?

Select all that apply.

☐ **1.** Fetal tone

☐ **2.** Fetal breathing

☐ **3.** Femur length

☐ **4.** Amniotic fluid volume

☐ **5.** Biparietal diameter

☐ **6.** Crown-rump length

Answer: 1, 2, 4

Rationale: A BPP is an ultrasound assessment of fetal well-being that includes the following components: nonstress test, fetal tone, fetal breathing, fetal motion, and volume of amniotic fluid. It's used to confirm the health of the fetus or identify abnormalities. Crown-rump length is used to assess gestational age during the first trimester. Biparietal diameter and femur length are also used to assess gestational age and are done in the second and third trimesters.

Nursing process step: Evaluation

Client needs category: Physiological integrity

Client needs subcategory: Reduction of risk potential

Cognitive level: Application

---

6. A nurse is performing a prenatal assessment on a client who is 32 weeks pregnant. She performs Leopold's maneuvers and determines that the fetus is in the cephalic position. Identify where the nurse should place the Doppler transducer to auscultate fetal heart tones.

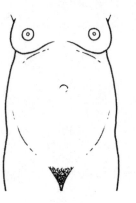

Answer:

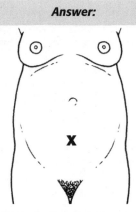

Rationale: When the fetus is in the cephalic position (head down), fetal heart tones are best auscultated midway between the symphysis pubis and the umbilicus. When the fetus is in the breech position, fetal heart tones are best heard at or above the level of the umbilicus.

Nursing process step: Assessment

Client needs category: Health promotion and maintenance

Client needs subcategory: None

Cognitive level: Analysis

7. A nurse is palpating the uterus of a client who is 20 weeks pregnant to measure fundal height. Identify the area on the abdomen where the nurse should expect to feel the uterine fundus.

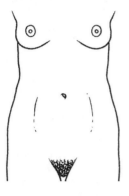

Answer:

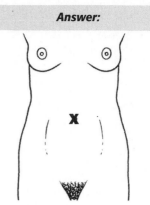

Rationale: At 20 weeks, the uterine fundus should be palpated approximately at the umbilicus. Fundal height should be measured from the symphysis pubis to the top of the uterus (McDonald's method). Serial measurements assess fetal growth over the course of the pregnancy. Between weeks 22 and 34, the number of centimeters measured correlate approximately with the week of gestation. However, if the woman is very tall or short, fundal height will differ.

Nursing process step: Assessment

Client needs category: Health promotion and maintenance

Client needs subcategory: None

Cognitive level: Application

---

8. A client who is 32 weeks pregnant is being monitored in the antepartum unit for pregnancy-induced hypertension. She suddenly complains of continuous abdominal pain and vaginal bleeding. Which of the following nursing interventions should be included in the care of this client?

Select all that apply.

- ☐ **1.** Evaluate maternal vital signs.
- ☐ **2.** Prepare for vaginal delivery.
- ☐ **3.** Reassure the client that she'll be able to continue the pregnancy.
- ☐ **4.** Auscultate fetal heart tones.
- ☐ **5.** Monitor the amount of vaginal bleeding.
- ☐ **6.** Monitor intake and output.

Answer: 1, 4, 5, 6

Rationale: The client's symptoms indicate that she's experiencing abruptio placentae. The nurse must immediately evaluate the mother's vital signs, auscultate fetal heart tones, monitor the amount of blood loss, and evaluate volume status by monitoring intake and output. After the severity of the abruption has been determined and blood and fluid have been replaced, a prompt cesarean (not vaginal) delivery is indicated if the fetus is in distress.

Nursing process step: Implementation

Client needs category: Physiological integrity

Client needs subcategory: Physiological adaptation

Cognitive level: Analysis

9. In early pregnancy, some clients complain of abdominal pain or pulling. Identify the area most commonly associated with this pain.

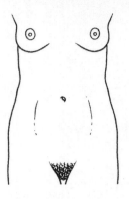

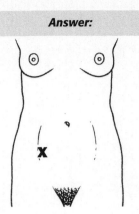

Rationale: As the uterus grows in early pregnancy, it deviates physically to the right. This shift, or dextrorotation, is due to the presence of the rectosigmoid colon in the left lower quadrant. As a result, many women complain of pain in the right lower quadrant.

Nursing process step: Evaluation

Client needs category: Health promotion and maintenance

Client needs subcategory: None

Cognitive level: Analysis

---

10. During a prenatal visit, a physician decides to admit a client to the hospital. Based on the nurse's admission note below, which complication of pregnancy would the physician suspect?

2/2/06 1100	30-year-old female admitted with nausea and vomiting. Pt. is 16 weeks pregnant and complains of thirst and vertigo. BP 120/70 mm Hg, RR 20, P 104, Temp 100° F. Pt. has had nothing to eat or drink for 24 hours. ———————————— S. Thomas, RN

☐ **1.** Iron-deficiency anemia

☐ **2.** Placenta previa

☐ **3.** Pregnancy-induced hypertension

☐ **4.** Hyperemesis gravidarum

Answer: 4

Rationale: Hyperemesis gravidarum is severe nausea and vomiting that persists after the first trimester. If untreated, it can lead to weight loss, starvation, dehydration, fluid and electrolyte imbalances, and acid-base disturbances. The client may report thirst, hiccups, oliguria, vertigo, and headache. A rapid pulse and elevated or subnormal temperature can also occur. Signs and symptoms of iron-deficiency anemia include fatigue, pallor, and exercise intolerance. Placenta previa causes painless, bright red, vaginal bleeding after 20 weeks of pregnancy. Pregnancy-induced hypertension usually develops after 20 weeks of pregnancy; the client reports sudden weight gain and presents with hypertension.

Nursing process step: Assessment

Client needs category: Physiological integrity

Client needs subcategory: Physiological adaptation

Cognitive level: Application

11. A pregnant client at 32 weeks' gestation has mild preeclampsia. She is discharged home with instructions to remain on bed rest. She should also be instructed to call her physician if she experiences which of the following symptoms?

Select all that apply.

☐ **1.** Headache

☐ **2.** Increased urine output

☐ **3.** Blurred vision

☐ **4.** Difficulty sleeping

☐ **5.** Epigastric pain

☐ **6.** Severe nausea and vomiting

Answer: 1, 3, 5, 6

Rationale: Headache, blurred vision, epigastric pain, and severe nausea and vomiting can indicate worsening preeclampsia. Decreased, not increased, urine output is a concern because preeclampsia is associated with decreased renal perfusion, leading to a reduction in the glomerular filtration rate and decreased urine output. Difficulty sleeping, a common complaint during the third trimester, is only a concern if it's caused by any of the other symptoms.

Nursing process step: Implementation

Client needs category: Physiological integrity

Client needs subcategory: Reduction of risk potential

Cognitive level: Application

12. A client who is 37 weeks pregnant comes to the office for a prenatal visit. A nurse performs Leopold's maneuvers to assess the position of the fetus. After performing the maneuvers, the nurse suspects that the physician will attempt external version. Where did the nurse palpate the head of the fetus?

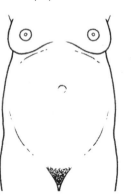

Answer:

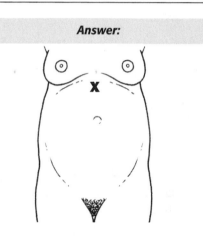

Rationale: If the fetal head is palpated at the top of the uterus, the fetus is in the breech position. That is, the head is not the presenting part and the physician may consider external version to convert the fetus to a vertex lie, or head-down position. This is accomplished by applying pressure on the maternal abdomen to turn the infant over, as in a somersault.

Nursing process step: Planning

Client needs category: Physiological integrity

Client needs subcategory: Reduction of risk potential

Cognitive level: Analysis

13. A nurse is teaching a course on the anatomy and physiology of reproduction. Identify the area where she should indicate that fertilization occurs.

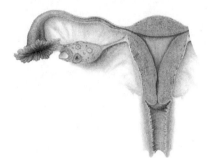

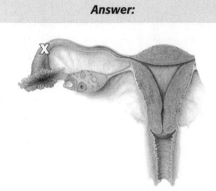

Rationale: After ejaculation, the sperm travel by flagellar movement through the cervical mucus into the fallopian tube to meet the descending ovum in the ampulla. Fertilization occurs in the ampulla (outer third) of the fallopian tube.

Nursing process step: Implementation

Client needs category: Health promotion and maintenance

Client needs subcategory: None

Cognitive level: Application

Intrapartum period

1. A nurse is evaluating a client who is 34 weeks pregnant for premature rupture of the membranes (PROM). Which findings indicate that PROM has occurred?

Select all that apply.

☐ **1.** Fernlike pattern when vaginal fluid is placed on a glass slide and allowed to dry

☐ **2.** Acidic pH of fluid when tested with nitrazine paper

☐ **3.** Presence of amniotic fluid in the vagina

☐ **4.** Cervical dilation of 6 cm

☐ **5.** Alkaline pH of fluid when tested with nitrazine paper

☐ **6.** Contractions occurring every 5 minutes

Answer: 1, 3, 5

Rationale: The fernlike pattern that occurs when vaginal fluid is placed on a glass slide and allowed to dry, the presence of amniotic fluid in the vagina, and an alkaline pH of fluid are all signs of ruptured membranes. The fernlike pattern is a result of the high sodium and protein content of the amniotic fluid. The presence of amniotic fluid in the vagina results from the expulsion of the fluid from the amniotic sac. Amniotic fluid tests as an alkaline fluid. Cervical dilation and regular contractions are signs of progressing labor but do not indicate PROM.

Nursing process step: Assessment

Client needs category: Physiological integrity

Client needs subcategory: Physiological adaptation

Cognitive level: Analysis

2. A client in the first stage of labor is being monitored using an external fetal monitor. After a nurse reviews the monitoring strip from the client's chart (shown below), into which of the following positions should she assist the client?

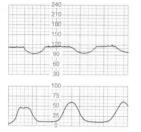

☐ **1.** Left lateral

☐ **2.** Right lateral

☐ **3.** Supine

☐ **4.** Prone

Answer: 1

Rationale: The fetal heart rate monitoring strip at left shows late decelerations, which indicate uteroplacental circulatory insufficiency and can lead to fetal hypoxia and acidosis if the underlying cause isn't corrected. The client should be turned onto her left side to increase placental perfusion and decrease contraction frequency. In addition, the I.V. fluid rate may be increased and oxygen administered. The right lateral, supine, and prone positions don't increase placental perfusion.

Nursing process step: Implementation

Client needs category: Physiological integrity

Client needs subcategory: Reduction of risk potential

Cognitive level: Analysis

---

3. On the waveform below, identify the area that indicates possible umbilical cord compression.

Answer:

Rationale: Variable decelerations are decreases in fetal heart rate that aren't related to the timing of contractions. They are characteristic of umbilical cord compression, which reduces blood flow between the placenta and fetus. These decelerations generally occur as drops of 10 to 60 beats/minute below the baseline.

Nursing process step: Assessment

Client needs category: Physiological integrity

Client needs subcategory: Reduction of risk potential

Cognitive level: Analysis

4. A client who is 29 weeks pregnant comes to the labor and delivery unit. She states that she's having contractions every 8 minutes. The client is also 3 cm dilated. Which of the following can the nurse expect to administer?

Select all that apply.

☐ **1.** Folic acid (Folvite)

☐ **2.** Terbutaline (Brethine)

☐ **3.** Betamethasone

☐ **4.** Rh$_O$ (D) immune globulin (Rhogam)

☐ **5.** I.V. fluids

☐ **6.** Meperidine (Demerol)

Answer: 2, 3, 5

Rationale: The client is at risk for preterm delivery. The nurse can expect that terbutaline, a beta-$_2$ agonist that relaxes smooth muscle, will be administered to halt contractions. The nurse can also expect that betamethasone, a corticosteroid, will be administered to decrease the risk of respiratory distress in the infant if preterm delivery occurs and that I.V. fluids will be given to expand the intravascular volume and decrease contractions if dehydration is the cause. Folic acid is a mineral recommended throughout pregnancy (especially in the first trimester) to decrease the risk of neural tube defects. It isn't used to address preterm delivery. Rh$_O$ (D) immune globulin is administered to Rh-negative clients who have been or are suspected of having been exposed to Rh-positive fetal blood. Meperidine is a narcotic used during labor and delivery to manage pain.

Nursing process step: Implementation

Client needs category: Physiological integrity

Client needs subcategory: Pharmacological and parenteral therapies

Cognitive level: Analysis

---

5. A nurse is monitoring a client who is receiving oxytocin (Pitocin) to induce labor. The nurse should observe for which of the following maternal adverse reactions?

Select all that apply.

☐ **1.** Hypertension

☐ **2.** Jaundice

☐ **3.** Dehydration

☐ **4.** Fluid overload

☐ **5.** Uterine tetany

☐ **6.** Bradycardia

Answer: 1, 4, 5

Rationale: Adverse effects of oxytocin in the mother include hypertension, fluid overload, uterine tetany, and tachycardia, not bradycardia. The antidiuretic effect of oxytocin increases renal reabsorption of water, leading to fluid overload — not dehydration. Jaundice and bradycardia are adverse reactions that may occur in the neonate.

Nursing process step: Assessment

Client needs category: Physiological integrity

Client needs subcategory: Pharmacological and parenteral therapies

Cognitive level: Application

6. A nurse is evaluating the external fetal monitoring strip (shown below) of a client who is in labor. Which of the following nursing interventions should the nurse implement?

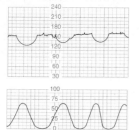

☐ **1.** Increase the I.V. fluid rate to boost intravascular volume.

☐ **2.** Reassure the client that the fetus isn't at risk and continue to monitor the fetal heart rate.

☐ **3.** Elevate the client's legs.

☐ **4.** Administer supplemental oxygen.

Answer: 2

Rationale: The monitoring strip from this client's chart shows early decelerations. These can result from head compression during normal labor and don't indicate fetal distress. The nurse should reassure the client and continue to monitor the fetal heart rate. The other nursing interventions aren't appropriate.

Nursing process step: Analysis

Client needs category: Health promotion and maintenance

Client needs subcategory: None

Cognitive level: Application

---

7. A client in labor is 8 cm dilated. The fetus, which is in vertex presentation, is 75% effaced and is at 0 station. In the illustration below, identify the level of the fetus's head.

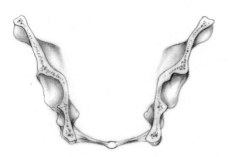

Answer:

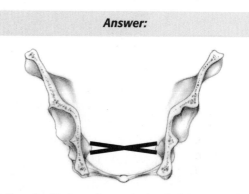

Rationale: Station refers to the level of the presenting part in relation to the pelvic inlet and the ischial spines. A 0 station indicates that the presenting part lies at the level of the ischial spines. Other stations are defined by their distance in centimeters above or below the ischial spines.

Nursing process step: Assessment

Client needs category: Health promotion and maintenance

Client needs subcategory: None

Cognitive level: Application

8. The nurse is evaluating a client's external fetal monitoring strip (shown below). Identify the area on this strip that causes her to be concerned about uteroplacental insufficiency.

Answer:

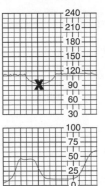

Rationale: This fetal monitoring strip illustrates a late deceleration. The decrease in fetal heart rate begins at the end of the contraction and does not return to baseline until the contraction is over. Late decelerations are caused by uteroplacental insufficiency resulting from decreased blood flow and oxygen transfer to the fetus through the intervillous spaces during uterine contractions.

Nursing process step: Assessment

Client needs category: Physiological integrity

Client needs subcategory: Reduction of risk potential

Cognitive level: Analysis

---

9. A nurse is caring for a client who's in the third stage of labor. The nurse knows that which of the following client behaviors are characteristic of this stage?

Select all that apply.

☐ **1.** The client is excited about the process.

☐ **2.** The client is focused on the neonate's condition.

☐ **3.** The client is exhausted from the labor process.

☐ **4.** The client states she has discomfort from uterine contractions.

☐ **5.** The client is apprehensive about the process.

Answer: 2, 4

Rationale: In the third stage of labor, the client focuses on the neonate's condition. Before the placenta is expelled, she may also state that she is experiencing discomfort from uterine contractions. Excitement and apprehension are characteristic of the first stage of labor. Exhaustion is common in the second stage of labor.

Nursing process step: Assessment

Client needs category: Psychosocial integrity

Client needs subcategory: None

Cognitive level: Application

10. A nurse is evaluating a fetal monitoring strip to time the contractions of a client in labor. Identify the beginning of the contraction in the illustration below.

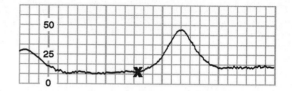

Answer:

Rationale: The beginning of a contraction, identified by a rise in pressure in the uterus, is indicated on the monitoring strip by movement of the waveform away from the baseline.

Nursing process step: Assessment

Client needs category: Health promotion and maintenance

Client needs subcategory: None

Cognitive level: Application

Postpartum period

1. A client has received treatment for a warm, reddened, painful area in the breast as well as cracked and fissured nipples. The client expresses the desire to continue breast-feeding. Which instructions should the nurse include to prevent a recurrence of this condition?

Select all that apply.

☐ **1.** Wash the nipples with soap and water.

☐ **2.** Change the breast pads frequently.

☐ **3.** Expose the nipples to air for part of each day.

☐ **4.** Wash hands before handling the breast and breast-feeding.

☐ **5.** Make sure that the baby grasps the nipple only.

☐ **6.** Release the baby's grasp on the nipple before removing the baby from the breast.

Answer: 2, 3, 4, 6

Rationale: To help prevent mastitis, an infection commonly associated with a break in the skin surface of the nipple, the nurse should suggest measures to prevent cracked and fissured nipples. Changing breast pads frequently and exposing the nipples to air for part of the day help keep the nipples dry and prevent irritation. Washing hands before handling the breast reduces the chance of accidentally introducing organisms into the breast. Releasing the baby's grasp on the nipple before removing the baby from the breast also reduces the chance of irritation. Nipples should be washed with water only; soap tends to remove the natural oils and increases the chance of cracking. The baby should grasp both the nipple and areola.

Nursing process step: Implementation

Client needs category: Health promotion and maintenance

Client needs subcategory: None

Cognitive level: Comprehension

2. A nurse is caring for a 1-day postpartum client. The progress note below informs, the nurse that the client is in which phase of the postpartum period?

5/24/05	Mother verbalizing labor and delivery
1715	experience. Doesn't appear confident about
	holding baby or changing diapers. Asking
	appropriate questions.——— J. Conners, RN

☐ **1.** Letting go

☐ **2.** Taking in

☐ **3.** Holding out

☐ **4.** Taking hold

Answer: 2

Rationale: The taking-in phase is normally the first postpartum phase. During this phase, the mother feels overwhelmed by the responsibilities of newborn care and is still fatigued from delivery. Taking hold is the next phase, when the client has rested and can learn mothering skills with confidence. Letting go is the final stage, when the client adapts to parenthood, her new role as a caregiver, and her new baby as a separate entity. Holding out isn't a valid phase.

Nursing process step: Assessment

Client needs category: Psychosocial integrity

Client needs subcategory: None

Cognitive level: Analysis

---

3. A nurse observes several interactions between a client and her neonate son. Which of the following behaviors of the mother would the nurse identify as evidence of mother-infant attachment?

Select all that apply.

☐ **1.** Talks to and coos at her son

☐ **2.** Cuddles her son close to her

☐ **3.** Doesn't make eye contact with her son

☐ **4.** Requests that the nurse take the baby to the nursery for feedings

☐ **5.** Encourages the father to hold the baby

☐ **6.** Takes a nap when the baby is sleeping

Answer: 1, 2

Rationale: Talking to, cooing at, and cuddling with her son are positive signs that the client is adapting to her new role as a mother. Eye contact, touching, and speaking help establish attachment with a neonate. Avoiding eye contact is a nonbonding behavior. Feeding a neonate is an important role of a new mother and facilitates attachment. Encouraging the father to hold the neonate will facilitate attachment between the neonate and his father. Resting while the neonate is sleeping will conserve needed energy and allow the mother to be alert and awake when her infant is awake; however, it isn't evidence of bonding.

Nursing process step: Evaluation

Client needs category: Psychosocial integrity

Client needs subcategory: None

Cognitive level: Analysis

4. A nurse is caring for a postpartum client suspected of developing postpartum psychosis. Which of the following statements accurately characterize this disorder?

Select all that apply.

☐ **1.** Symptoms start 2 days after delivery.

☐ **2.** The disorder is common in postpartum women.

☐ **3.** Symptoms include delusions and hallucinations.

☐ **4.** Suicide and infanticide are uncommon in this disorder.

☐ **5.** The disorder rarely occurs without a psychiatric history.

Answer: 3, 5

Rationale: A postpartum client should be suspected of psychosis if she exhibits delusions or hallucinations, generally starting within 4 weeks postpartum. Typically, the woman has a past history of a psychiatric disorder and treatment. A history of bipolar disorder is an important risk factor. The disorder occurs in less then 1% of postpartum mothers. It's considered a medical emergency. Suicide and infanticide are common.

Nursing process step: Assessment

Client needs category: Psychosocial integrity

Client needs subcategory: None

Cognitive level: Analysis

---

5. A mother with a history of varicose veins has just delivered her first baby. A nurse suspects that the mother has developed a pulmonary embolus. Which of the data below would lead to this nursing judgment?

Select all that apply.

☐ **1.** Sudden dyspnea

☐ **2.** Chills, fever

☐ **3.** Diaphoresis

☐ **4.** Hypertension

☐ **5.** Confusion

Answer: 1, 3, 5

Rationale: Sudden dyspnea with diaphoresis and confusion are classic signs and symptoms of a pulmonary embolus. In this disorder, a thrombus (stationary blood clot) dislodges from a varicose vein and becomes lodged in the pulmonary circulation. Chills and fever would indicate an infection. A client with an embolus could be hypotensive, not hypertensive.

Nursing process step: Assessment

Client needs category: Physiological integrity

Client needs subcategory: Physiological adaptation

Cognitive level: Analysis

6. A nurse is palpating the uterine fundus of a client who delivered a baby 8 hours ago. Identify the area where the nurse would expect to feel the fundus.

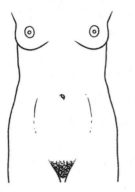

Answer:

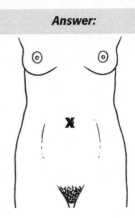

Rationale: The uterus should be felt at the level of the umbilicus from 1 hour to 24 hours after birth.

Nursing process step: Assessment

Client needs category: Physiological integrity

Client needs subcategory: Reduction of risk potential

Cognitive level: Application

---

7. A nurse is caring for a client in the fourth stage of labor. Based on the nurse's note below, which postpartum complication has the client developed?

6/7/05	Pt.'s 24-hour blood loss is 600 ml. Uterus is
1745	soft and relaxed on palpation and pt. has
	a full bladder. Assisted pt. in emptying
	bladder and notified Dr. G. McMann of
	findings. Vital signs stable at present. See
	graphic sheet for ongoing assessments and
	perineal pad weights.———— S. Jones, RN

☐ **1.** Postpartum hemorrhage

☐ **2.** Puerperal infection

☐ **3.** Deep vein thrombosis

☐ **4.** Mastitis

Answer: 1

Rationale: Blood loss from the uterus that exceeds 500 ml in a 24-hour period is considered postpartum hemorrhage. If uterine atony is the cause, the uterus feels soft and relaxed. A full bladder can prevent the uterus from contracting completely, increasing the risk of hemorrhage. Puerperal infection is an infection of the uterus and structures above; its characteristic sign is fever. Two major types of deep vein thrombosis occur in the postpartum period: pelvic and femoral. Each has different signs and symptoms, but both occur later in the postpartum period (femoral, after 10 days postpartum; pelvic, after 14 days). Mastitis is an inflammation of the mammary glands that disrupts normal lactation and usually develops 1 to 4 weeks postpartum.

Nursing process step: Assessment

Client needs category: Physiological integrity

Client needs subcategory: Reduction of risk potential

Cognitive level: Analysis

8. A nurse assesses a client's vaginal discharge on the first postpartum day and describes it in her progress note (shown below). Which of the following terms best describes the discharge?

3/30/06	Perineal pad changed two times this shift
1645	for moderate amount of red discharge.————
	——————————————— J. Jones, RN

☐ **1.** Lochia alba

☐ **2.** Lochia

☐ **3.** Lochia serosa

☐ **4.** Lochia rubra

Rationale: For the first 3 days after birth, the discharge is called *lochia rubra*. It consists almost entirely of blood, with only small particles of decidua and mucus. Lochia alba is a creamy white or colorless discharge that occurs 10 to 14 days postpartum. Lochia serosa is a pink or brownish discharge that occurs 4 to 14 days postpartum. The term *lochia* alone isn't a correct description of the discharge.

Nursing process step: Assessment

Client needs category: Physiological integrity

Client needs subcategory: Physiological adaptation

Cognitive level: Application

---

9. A home care lactation nurse has asked a client to keep a record of her intake, including calories, and output for 1 day. After reviewing the flow sheet that the client used to document the results (shown below), the nurse should make which of the following assessments?

Time period	Fluids (in ml)	Calories	Output (in ml)
7 a.m. to 11 a.m.	milk 240	breakfast 510	60
	orange juice 60		
11 a.m. to 3 p.m.	coffee 240	lunch 350	250
	orange juice 120	snack 80	200
	water 240		200
3 p.m. to 11 p.m.	water 240	dinner 500	100
	water 240	snack 350	230
	water 240		200
11 p.m. to 7 a.m.	water 240		300

☐ **1.** The client consumed an adequate amount of calories and fluids for breast-feeding.

☐ **2.** The client consumed an adequate amount of calories but not enough fluids for breast-feeding.

☐ **3.** The client consumed an adequate amount of fluids but not enough calories for breast-feeding.

☐ **4.** The client consumed an inadequate amount of fluids and calories for breast-feeding.

Rationale: New mothers who are breast-feeding should consume 2 to 3 L of fluids and 2,300 to 2,700 calories daily.

Nursing process step: Evaluation

Client needs category: Health promotion and maintenance

Client needs subcategory: None

Cognitive level: Analysis

The neonate

1. A nurse is doing a neurologic assessment on a 1-day-old neonate in the nursery. Which of the following findings would indicate possible asphyxia in utero?

Select all that apply.

☐ **1.** The neonate grasps the nurse's finger when she puts it in the palm of his hand.

☐ **2.** The neonate does stepping movements when held upright with the sole of his foot touching a surface.

☐ **3.** The neonate's toes don't curl downward when the soles of his feet are touched.

☐ **4.** The neonate doesn't respond when the nurse claps her hands above him.

☐ **5.** The neonate turns toward the nurse's finger when she touches his cheek.

☐ **6.** The neonate displays weak, ineffective sucking.

Answer: 3, 4, 6

Rationale: If the neonate's toes don't curl downward when the soles of his feet are touched and he doesn't respond to a loud sound, neurologic damage from asphyxia may have occurred. A normal neurologic response would be the toes curling downward with touching and the arms and legs extending with a loud noise. Weak, ineffective sucking is another sign of neurologic damage. A neonate should grasp a person's finger when it's placed in the palm of his hand, do stepping movements when held upright with the sole of foot touching a surface, and turn toward the nurse's finger when she touches his cheek.

Nursing process step: Assessment

Client needs category: Health promotion and maintenance

Client needs subcategory: None

Cognitive level: Application

---

2. What information should the nurse include when teaching postcircumcision care to parents of a neonate prior to discharge from the hospital?

Select all that apply.

☐ **1.** The infant must void before being discharged home.

☐ **2.** Petroleum jelly or antibiotic ointment should be applied to the glans of the penis with each diaper change.

☐ **3.** The infant can have tub baths while the circumcision heals.

☐ **4.** Any amount of blood noted on the front of the diaper should be reported.

☐ **5.** The circumcision will require care for 2 to 4 days after discharge.

Answer: 1, 2, 5

Rationale: The infant must void prior to discharge to ensure that the urethra isn't obstructed. A lubricating or antibiotic ointment should be applied with each diaper change. Typically, the penis heals within 2 to 4 days, and circumcision care is needed for that period only. To prevent infection, the infant should not have tub baths until the circumcision is healed; sponge baths are appropriate. A small amount of bleeding is expected following a circumcision; parents should report only a large amount of bleeding.

Nursing process step: Implementation

Client needs category: Safe, effective care environment

Client needs subcategory: Management of care

Cognitive level: Application

3. A 14-day-old neonate is admitted for aspiration pneumonia. The results of a barium swallow confirm a diagnosis of gastroesophageal reflux with resulting aspiration pneumonia. Identify the area of the stomach associated with this diagnosis.

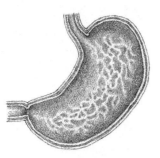

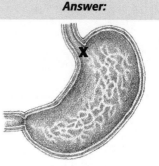

Rationale: Gastroesophageal reflux is a neuromotor disturbance in which the cardiac sphincter located between the stomach and the esophagus is weak. This allows easy regurgitation of gastric contents into the esophagus, causing possible aspiration into the lungs.

Nursing process step: Analysis

Client needs category: Physiological integrity

Client needs subcategory: Physiological adaptation

Cognitive level: Application

---

4. A nurse is demonstrating cord care to a mother of a neonate. Which actions would the nurse teach the mother to perform?

Select all that apply.

☐ **1.** Keep the diaper below the cord.

☐ **2.** Tug gently on the cord as it begins to dry.

☐ **3.** Apply antibiotic ointment to the cord twice daily.

☐ **4.** Only sponge-bathe the infant until the cord falls off.

☐ **5.** Clean the length of the cord with alcohol several times daily.

☐ **6.** Wash the cord with mild soap and water.

Answer: 1, 4, 5

Rationale: The diaper should be positioned below the cord to allow it to air-dry and to prevent urine from getting on the cord. The nurse should instruct the parents to sponge-bathe the infant until the cord falls off. Soap and water should not be used as a part of cord care. The entire cord should be cleaned with alcohol, using a cotton swab or another appropriate method, several times a day. Parents should also be instructed to never pull on the cord, but to allow it to fall off naturally. Antibiotic ointments are contraindicated unless there are signs of infection.

Nursing process step: Implementation

Client needs category: Safe, effective care environment

Client needs subcategory: Safety and infection control

Cognitive level: Application

5. At 5 minutes of age, a neonate is pink with acrocyanosis; has flexed knees, clinched fists, a whimpering cry, and a heart rate of 128 beats/minute; and withdraws his foot when slapped on the sole. What 5-minute Apgar score would the nurse record for this neonate?

Sign	Apgar Score		
	0	1	2
Heart rate	Absent	Less than 100 beats/minute (slow)	More than 100 beats/minute
Respiratory effort	Absent	Slow, irregular	Good cry
Muscle tone	Flaccid	Some flexion and resistance to extension of extremities	Active motion
Reflex irritability	No response	Grimace or weak cry	Vigorous cry
Color	Pallor, cyanosis	Pink body, blue extremities	Completely pink

Answer: 8

Rationale: The Apgar score assesses a neonate immediately after birth and at 5 minutes of age for heart rate, respiratory effort, muscle tone, reflex irritability, and color. Each function is scored from zero (poor) to 2 (normal). This neonate has a heart rate above 100 beats/minute (score of 2); a weak cry (score of 1); good flexion (score of 2); a good response to a slap on the sole (score of 2); and pink color with acrocyanosis (score of 1). Thus, his total Apgar score is 8.

Nursing process step: Assessment

Client needs category: Physiological integrity

Client needs subcategory: Physiological adaptation

Cognitive level: Analysis

6. A nurse is administering vitamin K (AquaMEPHYTON) to a neonate following delivery. The medication comes in a concentration of 2 mg/ml, and the ordered dose is 0.5 mg to be given subcutaneously. How many milliliters should the nurse administer?

Answer: 0.25

Rationale: Use the following formula to calculate drug dosages:

Dose on hand/Quantity on hand = Dose desired/X

2 mg/ml = 0.5 mg/X

X = 0.25 ml.

Nursing process step: Planning

Client needs category: Physiological integrity

Client needs subcategory: Pharmacological and parenteral therapies

Cognitive level: Analysis

7. A nurse is eliciting reflexes in a neonate during a physical examination. Identify the area that the nurse would touch to elicit a plantar grasp reflex.

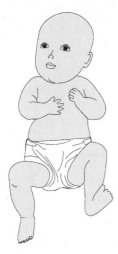

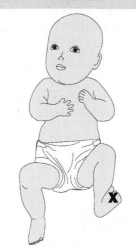

Rationale: To elicit a plantar grasp reflex, the nurse should touch the sole of the foot near the base of the digits, causing flexion or grasping. This reflex disappears at around age 9 months.

Nursing process step: Assessment

Client needs category: Health promotion and maintenance

Client needs subcategory: None

Cognitive level: Application

8. A nurse is providing care to a neonate. Place the following steps in the order that the nurse should implement them to properly perform ophthalmia neonatorum prophylaxis.

1.	Close and manipulate the eyelids to spread the medication over the eye.
2.	Shield the neonate's eyes from direct light, and tilt his head slightly to the side that will receive the treatment.
3.	Repeat the procedure for the other eye.
4.	Wash the hands and put on gloves.
5.	Instill the ointment in the lower conjunctival sac.
6.	Gently raise the neonate's upper eyelid with the index finger, and pull the lower eyelid down with the thumb.

Answer:

4.	Wash the hands and put on gloves.
2.	Shield the neonate's eyes from direct light, and tilt his head slightly to the side that will receive the treatment.
6.	Gently raise the neonate's upper eyelid with the index finger, and pull the lower eyelid down with the thumb.
5.	Instill the ointment in the lower conjunctival sac.
1.	Close and manipulate the eyelids to spread the medication over the eye.
3.	Repeat the procedure for the other eye.

Rationale: Ophthalmia neonatorum prophylaxis is the instillation of 0.5% erythromycin or 1% tetracycline ointment into a neonate's eyes. This procedure is performed to prevent gonorrheal and chlamydial conjunctivitis. All 50 states mandate that this treatment be given within 1 hour of birth to decrease the risk of permanent eye damage and blindness.

Nursing process step: Assessment

Client needs category: Physiological integrity

Client needs subcategory: Physiological adaptation

Cognitive level: Application

PART | FOUR

Pediatric nursing

The infant

1. A physician orders an I.V. infusion of dextrose 5% in quarter-normal saline solution to be infused at 7 ml/kg/hr for a 10-month-old infant. The infant weighs 22 lb. How many milligrams of the ordered solution should the nurse infuse each hour?

_____

Answer: 70

Rationale: To perform this dosage calculation, the nurse should first convert the infant's weight to kilograms:

$$2.2 \text{ lb/kg} = 22 \text{ lb/X kg}$$

$$X = 22 \div 2.2$$

$$X = 10 \text{ kg.}$$

Next, she should multiply the infant's weight by the ordered rate:

$$10 \text{ kg} \times 7 \text{ ml/kg/hr} = 70 \text{ ml/hr.}$$

Nursing process step: Implementation

Client needs category: Physiological integrity

Client needs subcategory: Pharmacological and parenteral therapies

Cognitive level: Application

---

2. A nurse is teaching the parents of a 6-month-old infant about normal growth and development. Which of the following statements is true regarding infant development?

Select all that apply.

☐ **1.** A 6-month-old infant has difficulty holding objects.

☐ **2.** A 6-month-old infant can usually roll from prone to supine and supine to prone positions.

☐ **3.** A teething ring is appropriate for a 6-month-old infant.

☐ **4.** Stranger anxiety usually peaks at age 12 to 18 months.

☐ **5.** Head lag is commonly noted in infants at age 6 months.

☐ **6.** Lack of visual coordination usually resolves by age 6 months.

Answer: 2, 3, 6

Rationale: Gross motor skills of the 6-month-old infant include rolling from front to back and back to front. Teething usually begins around age 6 months and, therefore, a teething ring is appropriate. Visual coordination is usually resolved by age 6 months. At age 6 months, fine motor skills include purposeful grasping and releasing of objects and transferring objects from one hand to another. Stranger anxiety normally peaks at 8 months. The 6-month-old infant also should have good head control and no longer display head lag when pulled up to a sitting position.

Nursing process step: Implementation

Client needs category: Health promotion and maintenance

Client needs subcategory: None

Cognitive level: Application

3. An infant who weighs 8 kg is to receive ampicillin (Omnipen) 25 mg/kg I.V. every 6 hours. How many milligrams should a nurse administer per dose?

_____

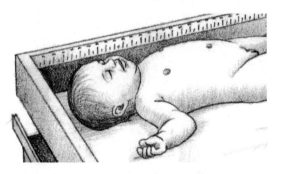

4. A nurse is conducting a physical examination on an infant. Identify the anatomic landmark she should use to measure chest circumference.

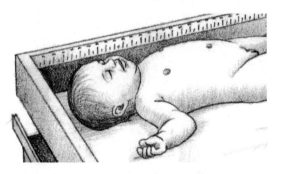

Answer: 200

Rationale: The nurse should calculate the correct dose by multiplying the infant's weight by the ordered rate:

$$8 \text{ kg} \times 25 \text{ mg/kg} = 200 \text{ mg}$$

Nursing process step: Implementation

Client needs category: Physiological integrity

Client needs subcategory: Pharmacological and parenteral therapies

Cognitive level: Application

Answer:

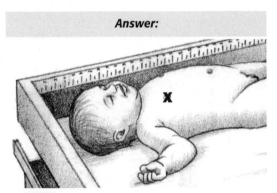

Rationale: Chest circumference is most accurately measured by placing the measuring tape around the infant's nipples. Measuring above or below the nipples will yield a false measurement. The measurement should be taken after exhalation.

Nursing process step: Assessment

Client needs category: Health promotion and maintenance

Client needs subcategory: None

Cognitive level: Application

5. A healthy 2-month-old infant is being seen in the local clinic for a well-child checkup and his initial immunizations. A nurse should anticipate administering which immunizations?

Select all that apply.

☐ **1.** DTaP (diphtheria, tetanus, and acellular pertussis)

☐ **2.** MMR (measles, mumps, and rubella)

☐ **3.** OPV (oral polio vaccine)

☐ **4.** HBV (hepatitis B vaccine)

☐ **5.** Varicella zoster (chickenpox) vaccine

☐ **6.** HIB (*Haemophilus influenzae* vaccine)

☐ **7.** Pneumococcal vaccine

Answer: 1, 4, 6, 7

Rationale: At age 2 months, the American Academy of Pediatrics recommends the administration of DTaP, IPV (inactivated polio vaccine), HBV, HIB, and pneumococcal vaccine. The MMR immunization should be administered at 12 to 15 months. The IPV — not the OPV — is currently used to minimize spread of the disease. The varicella zoster vaccine may be given any time after the child's first birthday.

Nursing process step: Implementation

Client needs category: Health promotion and maintenance

Client needs subcategory: None

Cognitive level: Application

---

6. When assessing an infant for changes in intracranial pressure (ICP), it's important to palpate the fontanels. Identify the area where a nurse should palpate to assess the anterior fontanel.

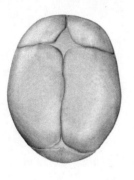

Answer:

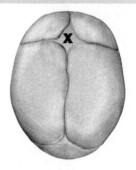

Rationale: The anterior fontanel is formed by the junction of the sagittal, frontal, and coronal sutures. It's shaped like a diamond and normally measures 4 to 5 cm at its widest point. A widened, bulging fontanel is a sign of increased ICP.

Nursing process step: Assessment

Client needs category: Health promotion and maintenance

Client needs subcategory: None

Cognitive level: Application

7. A parent is planning to enroll her 9-month-old infant in a day care facility. The parent asks a nurse what to look for as indicators that the facility is adhering to good infection control measures. How should the nurse reply?

Select all that apply.

☐ **1.** The facility keeps boxes of gloves in the director's office.

☐ **2.** Soiled diapers are discarded in covered receptacles.

☐ **3.** Toys are kept on the floor for the children to share.

☐ **4.** Disposable papers are used on the diaper-changing surfaces.

☐ **5.** Facilities for handwashing are located in every classroom.

☐ **6.** Soiled clothing and cloth diapers are sent home in labeled paper bags.

Rationale: A parent can assess infection control measures by appraising steps taken by the facility to prevent the spread of diseases. Placing soiled diapers in covered receptacles, covering the diaper-changing surfaces with disposable papers, and ensuring that sinks are available for personnel to wash their hands after activities are all indicators that infection control measures are being followed. Gloves should be readily available to personnel and, therefore, should be kept in every room—not in an office. Toys typically are shared by numerous children; however, this contributes to the spread of germs and infections. All soiled clothing and cloth diapers should be placed in a sealed plastic bag before being sent home.

Nursing process step: Implementation

Client needs category: Safe, effective care environment

Client needs subcategory: Safety and infection control

Cognitive level: Application

---

8. A nurse is performing cardiopulmonary resuscitation (CPR) on an infant. Identify the area where the nurse should assess for a pulse.

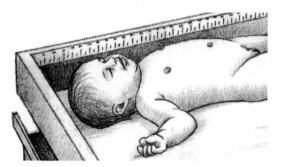

Answer:

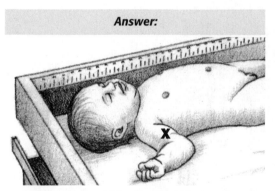

Rationale: The brachial pulse should be used to assess for a pulse when performing infant CPR. The carotid pulse, which is used in children and adults, is extremely difficult to locate in an infant because of his short neck.

Nursing process step: Assessment

Client needs category: Physiological adaptation

Client needs subcategory: Physiological integrity

Cognitive level: Application

9. A nurse is assessing a 10-month-old infant during a checkup. Which developmental milestones would the nurse expect the infant to display?

Select all that apply.

☐ **1.** Holding head erect

☐ **2.** Self-feeding

☐ **3.** Demonstrating good bowel and bladder control

☐ **4.** Sitting on a firm surface without support

☐ **5.** Bearing the majority of weight on legs

☐ **6.** Walking alone

Answer: 1, 4, 5

Rationale: By age 4 months, an infant should be able to hold his head erect. By age 9 months, the infant should be able to sit on a firm surface without support and bear the majority of weight on his legs (for example, walking while holding on to furniture). Self-feeding and bowel and bladder control are developmental milestones of toddlers. By age 12 months, the infant should be able to stand on his own and may take his first steps.

Nursing process step: Assessment

Client needs category: Health promotion and maintenance

Client needs subcategory: None

Cognitive level: Application

---

10. A nurse is conducting an infant nutrition class for parents. Which of the following foods should the nurse tell parents that they may introduce during the first year of life?

Select all that apply.

☐ **1.** Sliced beef

☐ **2.** Pureed fruits

☐ **3.** Whole milk

☐ **4.** Rice cereal

☐ **5.** Strained vegetables

☐ **6.** Fruit juice

Answer: 2, 4, 5

Rationale: The first food provided to a neonate is breast milk or formula. Between ages 4 and 6 months, rice cereal can be introduced, followed by pureed or strained fruits and vegetables, then strained or ground meat. Meats must be chopped or ground before they're fed to an infant to prevent choking. Infants should not be given whole milk until they're at least 1 year old. Fruit drinks provide no nutritional benefit and shouldn't be encouraged.

Nursing process step: Implementation

Client needs category: Health promotion and maintenance

Client needs subcategory: None

Cognitive level: Application

The toddler

1. A nurse is preparing a dose of amoxicillin for a 3-year-old with acute otitis media. The child weighs 33 lb. The dosage prescribed is 50 mg/kg/day in divided doses every 8 hours. The concentration of the drug is 250 mg/5 ml. How many milliliters should the nurse administer?

Answer: 5

Rationale: To calculate the child's weight in kilograms, the nurse should use the following formula:

$$2.2 \text{ lb}/1 \text{ kg} = 33 \text{ lb}/X \text{ kg}$$

$$X = 33 \div 2.2$$

$$X = 15 \text{ kg}.$$

Next, the nurse should calculate the daily dosage for the child:

$$50 \text{ mg/kg/day} \times 15 \text{ kg} = 750 \text{ mg/day}.$$

To determine divided daily dosage, the nurse should know that "every 8 hours" means 3 times per day. So, she should perform that calculation in this way:

$$\text{Total daily dosage} \div 3 \text{ times per day} = \text{Divided daily dosage}$$

$$750 \text{ mg/day} \div 3 = 250 \text{ mg}.$$

The drug's concentration is 250 mg/5 ml, so the nurse should administer 5 ml.

Nursing process step: Implementation

Client needs category: Physiological integrity

Client needs subcategory: Pharmacological and parenteral therapies

Cognitive level: Application

---

2. A 3-year-old is to receive 500 ml of dextrose 5% in normal saline solution over 8 hours. At what rate (in milliliters per hour) should a nurse set the infusion pump?

Answer: 62.5

Rationale: To calculate the rate per hour for the infusion, the nurse should divide 500 ml by 8 hours:

$$500 \text{ ml} \div 8 \text{ hours} = 62.5 \text{ ml/hour}.$$

Nursing process step: Implementation

Client needs category: Physiological integrity

Client needs subcategory: Pharmacological and parenteral therapies

Cognitive level: Application

3. A 2½-year-old is being treated for pneumonia. After reviewing the respiratory section of the client care flow sheet (shown below), a nurse concludes that she should place the child in which position to maximize oxygenation?

Date: 4/2/06	2300-0700	0700-1500	1500-2300
Breath sounds	Diminished BS LLL	Diminished BS LLL	Crackles LLL
Treatment/results	-----------	CPT & postural drainage	CPT & postural drainage
Cough/results	Nonproductive	Nonproductive	Yellow sputum
Oxygen therapy	Humidifier	Humidifier	Humidifier

☐ **1.** Left side

☐ **2.** Right side

☐ **3.** Supine

☐ **4.** Supine with the head of the bed elevated 30 degrees

Answer: 2

Rationale: The client should be positioned on his right side. Gravity will contribute to mobilizing secretions from the affected (left) lung, therefore allowing for improved blood flow and oxygenation.

Nursing process step: Implementation

Client needs category: Physiological integrity

Client needs subcategory: Physiological adaptation

Cognitive level: Analysis

---

4. A 15-month-old has just received his routine immunizations, including diphtheria, tetanus, and acellular pertussis (DTaP); inactivated polio vaccine (IPV); and measles, mumps, and rubella (MMR). What information should the nurse give to the parents before they leave the office?

Select all that apply.

☐ **1.** Minor symptoms can be treated with acetaminophen (Tylenol).

☐ **2.** Minor symptoms can be treated with aspirin.

☐ **3.** Call the office if the toddler develops a fever above 103° F (39.4° C), seizures, or difficulty breathing.

☐ **4.** Soreness at the immunization site and mild fever are common.

☐ **5.** The immunizations prevent the toddler from contracting their associated diseases.

☐ **6.** The toddler should restrict his activity for the remainder of the day.

Answer: 1, 3, 4

Rationale: Minor symptoms, such as soreness at the immunization site and mild fever, can be treated with acetaminophen or ibuprofen. Aspirin should be avoided in children because of its association with Reye's syndrome. The parents should notify the clinic if serious complications (such as a fever above 103° F, seizures, or difficulty breathing) occur. Minor discomforts, such as soreness and mild fever, are common after immunizations. Immunizing the child decreases the health risks associated with contracting certain diseases; it doesn't prevent the toddler from acquiring them. Although the child may prefer to rest after immunizations, it isn't necessary to restrict his activity.

Nursing process step: Implementation

Client needs category: Health promotion and maintenance

Client needs subcategory: None

Cognitive level: Application

5. A nurse is feeling the apical impulse of a 28-month-old child. Identify the area where the nurse should assess the apical impulse.

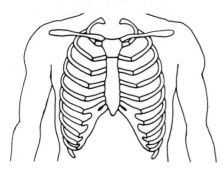

Answer:

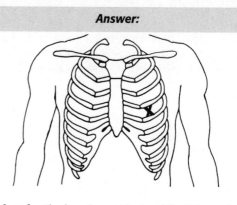

Rationale: The heart's apex for a toddler is located at the fourth intercostal space immediately to the left of the midclavicular line. It's one or two intercostal spaces above what's considered normal for an adult because the heart's position in a child of this age is more horizontal and larger in diameter than that of an adult.

Nursing process step: Assessment

Client needs category: Health promotion and maintenance

Client needs subcategory: None

Cognitive level: Application

---

6. A nurse is caring for a 3-year-old with viral meningitis. Which signs and symptoms would the nurse expect to find during the initial assessment?

Select all that apply.

☐ **1.** Bulging anterior fontanel

☐ **2.** Fever

☐ **3.** Nuchal rigidity

☐ **4.** Petechiae

☐ **5.** Irritability

☐ **6.** Photophobia

☐ **7.** Hypothermia

Answer: 2, 3, 5, 6

Rationale: Common signs and symptoms of viral meningitis include fever, nuchal rigidity, irritability, and photophobia. A bulging anterior fontanel is a sign of hydrocephalus, which isn't likely to occur in a toddler because the anterior fontanel typically closes by age 24 months. A petechial, purpuric rash may be seen with bacterial meningitis. Hypothermia is a common sign of bacterial meningitis in an infant younger than age 3 months.

Nursing process step: Assessment

Client needs category: Physiological integrity

Client needs subcategory: Physiological adaptation

Cognitive level: Application

7. A 3-year-old is being treated for severe status asthmaticus. After reviewing the progress notes (shown below), a nurse should determine that this client is being treated for which of the following conditions?

4/5/06 0600	Pt. was acutely restless, diaphoretic, and with SOB at 0530. Dr. T. Smith notified and ordered ABG analysis. ABG drawn from R radial artery. Stat results as follows: pH 7.28, Paco₂ 55 mm Hg, HCO₃⁻ 26 mEq/L. Dr. Smith with pt. now. ————J. Collins, RN.

☐ **1.** Metabolic acidosis

☐ **2.** Respiratory alkalosis

☐ **3.** Respiratory acidosis

☐ **4.** Metabolic alkalosis

Answer: 3

Rationale: A pH less than 7.35 and a partial pressure of arterial carbon dioxide ($Paco_2$) greater than 45 mm Hg indicate respiratory acidosis. Status asthmaticus is a medical emergency characterized by respiratory distress. At first, the client hyperventilates; then respiratory alkalosis occurs, followed by metabolic acidosis. If treatment is ineffective or hasn't started, symptoms can progress to hypoventilation and respiratory acidosis, which are life-threatening. A client with respiratory alkalosis would have a pH greater than 7.45 and a $Paco_2$ less than 35 mm Hg. Metabolic acidosis is characterized by a pH less than 7.35 and a bicarbonate (HCO_3^-) level less than 22mEq/L. Metabolic alkalosis is characterized by a pH greater than 7.45 and HCO_3^- above 26 mEq/L.

Nursing process step: Analysis

Client needs subcategory: Physiological integrity

Client needs subcategory: Physiological adaptation

Cognitive level: Analysis

---

8. A 30-month-old toddler is being evaluated for a ventricular septal defect (VSD). Identify the area where a VSD occurs.

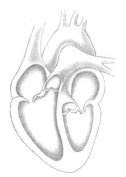

Answer:

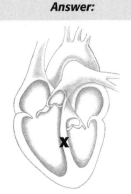

Rationale: A VSD is a small hole between the right and left ventricles that allows blood to shunt between them, causing right ventricular hypertrophy and, if left untreated, biventricular heart failure. It's a common congenital heart defect and accounts for 20% to 30% of all heart lesions.

Nursing process step: Assessment

Client needs category: Physiological integrity

Client needs subcategory: Physiological adaptation

Cognitive level: Application

9. A child weighing 44 lb is to receive 45 mg/kg/day of penicillin V potassium oral suspension in four divided doses every 6 hours. The suspension that's available is penicillin V potassium 125 mg/5 ml. How many milliliters should the nurse administer for each dose?

_____

Answer: 9

Rationale: First convert the child's weight to kilograms:

$$44 \text{ lb} \div 2.2 \text{ kg/lb} = 20 \text{ kg}.$$

Next, determine the daily dose:

$$45 \text{ mg:1kg} = X \text{ mg:20 kg}$$

$$45 \times 20 = 1 \times X$$

$$900 = X.$$

Then determine the dose to administer every 6 hours (4 doses):

$$900 \text{ mg} \div 4 = 225 \text{ mg}.$$

Finally, determine the volume to be given for each dose:

$$225 \text{ mg:X} = 125 \text{ mg:5 ml}$$

$$1125 \text{ mg/ml} = 125 \text{ mg/X}$$

$$9 \text{ ml} = X.$$

Nursing process step: Implementation

Client needs category: Physiological integrity

Client needs subcategory: Pharmacological and parenteral therapies

Cognitive level: Application

The preschooler

1. A 4½-year-old is ordered to receive 25 ml/hour of I.V. solution. The nurse is using a pediatric microdrip chamber to administer the medication. For how many drops per minute should the microdrip chamber be set?

_____

Answer: 25

Rationale: When using a pediatric microdrip chamber, the number of milliliters per hour equals the number of drops per minute. If 25 ml/hour is ordered, the I.V. solution should infuse at 25 drops/minute.

Nursing process step: Implementation

Client needs category: Physiological integrity

Client needs subcategory: Pharmacological and parenteral therapies

Cognitive level: Application

2. A 44-lb preschooler is being treated for inflammation. The physician orders 0.2 mg/kg/day of dexamethasone (Decadron) by mouth to be administered every 6 hours. The elixir comes in a strength of 0.5 mg/5 ml. How many milliliters of dexamethasone should a nurse give this client per dose?

_____

Rationale: To perform this dosage calculation, the nurse should first convert the child's weight from pounds to kilograms:

$$44 \text{ lb} \div 2.2 \text{ lb/kg} = 20 \text{ kg.}$$

Then she should calculate the total daily dose for the child:

$$20 \text{ kg} \times 0.2 \text{ mg/kg/day} = 4 \text{ mg.}$$

Next, the nurse should calculate the amount to be given at each dose:

$$4 \text{ mg} \div 4 \text{ doses} = 1 \text{ mg/dose.}$$

The available elixir contains 0.5 mg of drug per 5 ml. Therefore, to give 1 mg of the drug, the nurse should administer 10 ml to the child for each dose.

Nursing process step: Implementation

Client needs category: Physiological integrity

Client needs subcategory: Pharmacological and parenteral therapies

Cognitive level: Analysis

---

3. A nurse is performing a Denver Developmental Screening Test II on a 4½-year-old child. What behaviors should the nurse expect the child to demonstrate?

Select all that apply.

☐ **1.** He balances on each foot for at least 6 seconds.

☐ **2.** He copies a square that has straight lines and square corners.

☐ **3.** He prepares his own cereal without help.

☐ **4.** He copies a circle that's closed or very nearly closed.

☐ **5.** He speaks clearly.

☐ **6.** He draws a person with at least three body parts.

Rationale: By age 4½, a child should be able to prepare a bowl of cereal without help, copy a circle, speak clearly, and draw a person with at least three body parts. The majority of children don't achieve balancing on each foot for 6 seconds until about age 5½. Less than 25% of all children are able to correctly copy a square by age 4.

Nursing process step: Analysis

Client needs category: Health promotion and maintenance

Client needs subcategory: None

Cognitive level: Analysis

4. A 4-year-old child has recently been diagnosed with acute lymphocytic leukemia (ALL). What information about ALL should a nurse provide when educating the child's parents?

Select all that apply.

☐ **1.** ALL is a rare form of childhood leukemia.

☐ **2.** ALL affects all blood-forming organs and systems throughout the body.

☐ **3.** Because of the increased risk of bleeding, the child shouldn't brush his teeth.

☐ **4.** Adverse effects of treatment include sleepiness, alopecia, and stomatitis.

☐ **5.** There's a 95% chance of obtaining remission with treatment.

☐ **6.** The child shouldn't be disciplined during this difficult time.

Answer: 2, 4, 5

Rationale: In ALL, immature white blood cells (WBCs) crowd out healthy WBCs, red blood cells, and platelets in the bone marrow. These abnormal WBCs affect all blood-forming organs and systems. Common adverse effects of chemotherapy and radiation include nausea, vomiting, diarrhea, sleepiness, alopecia, anemia, stomatitis, pain, and increased susceptibility to infection. Remission occur in 95% of cases. Brushing teeth does not produce bleeding. A child with leukemia still needs appropriate discipline and limits. A lack of consistent parenting may lead to negative behaviors and fear.

Nursing process step: Implementation

Client needs category: Physiological integrity

Client needs subcategory: Reduction of risk potential

Cognitive level: Application

---

5. A critically ill 4-year-old is in the pediatric intensive care unit. Telemetry monitoring reveals junctional tachycardia. Identify where this arrhythmia originates.

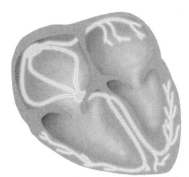

Answer:

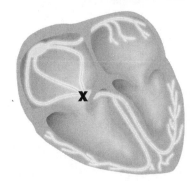

Rationale: In junctional tachycardia, the atrioventricular node fires rapidly. The atria are depolarized by retrograde conduction; however, conduction through the ventricles remains normal.

Nursing process step: Assessment

Client needs category: Physiological integrity

Client needs subcategory: Physiological adaptation

Cognitive level: Analysis

6. A school nurse is conducting registration for a first-grader. Which of the following immunizations should the school nurse verify that the child has had?

Select all that apply.

☐ **1.** Hepatitis B series

☐ **2.** Diphtheria-tetanus-pertussis series

☐ **3.** *Haemophilus influenzae* type b series

☐ **4.** Varicella zoster

☐ **5.** Pneumonia vaccine

☐ **6.** Oral polio series

Answer: 1, 2, 3

Rationale: Hepatitis B series, diphtheria-tetanus-pertussis series, *Haemophilus influenzae* type b series, and inactivated, not oral, polio series are the immunizations that the child should receive before entering first grade. The oral polio vaccine was discontinued; the safer inactivated polio vaccine is now used. The varicella zoster vaccine is administered only if the child hasn't had chickenpox. Some states require proof of vaccination if the child hasn't had chickenpox and is not required in all states. Pneumonia vaccine isn't required or routinely given to children.

Nursing process step: Analysis

Client needs category: Physiological integrity

Client needs subcategory: Physiological adaptation

Cognitive level: Analysis

---

7. A 4-year-old child is brought to the emergency department in cardiac arrest. The staff performs cardiopulmonary resuscitation (CPR). Identify the area where the child's pulse should be checked.

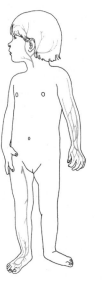

Answer:

Rationale: The carotid artery should be used to check for a pulse when performing CPR on children and adults. The brachial pulse should be used when performing CPR on an infant.

Nursing process step: Assessment

Client needs category: Physiological integrity

Client needs subcategory: Physiological adaptation

Cognitive level: Application

8. A preschooler is scheduled to have a Wilms' tumor removed. Identify the area of the urinary system where this tumor is located.

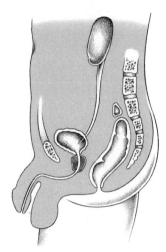

Answer:

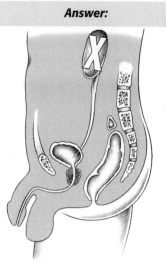

Rationale: A Wilms' tumor, also known as a nephroblastoma, is located on the kidney. The most common intra-abdominal tumor in children, Wilms' tumor usually affects children ages 2 to 4 and favors the left kidney.

Nursing process step: Assessment

Client needs category: Physiological integrity

Client needs subcategory: Physiological adaptation

Cognitive level: Application

---

9. A nurse is caring for a 5-year-old who is in the terminal stages of cancer. Which statements are true?

Select all that apply.

☐ **1.** The parents may be at different stages of grief in dealing with the child's impending death.

☐ **2.** The child is thinking about the future and knows he may not be able to participate.

☐ **3.** The dying child may become clingy and act like a toddler.

☐ **4.** Whispering in the child's room will help the child to cope.

☐ **5.** The death of a child may have long-term disruptive effects on the family.

☐ **6.** The child doesn't fully understand the concept of death.

Answer: 1, 3, 5, 6

Rationale: When dealing with a dying child, parents may be at different stages of grief at different times. The child may regress in his behaviors. The stress of a child's death commonly results in divorce and behavioral problems in siblings. Preschoolers see illness and death as a form of punishment. They fear separation from parents and might worry about who will provide care for them. Preschoolers have only a rudimentary concept of time; thinking about the future is typical of an adolescent facing death, not a preschooler. Whispering in front of the child only increases his fear of death.

Nursing process step: Analysis

Client needs category: Psychosocial integrity

Client needs subcategory: None

Cognitive level: Analysis

1. A 7-year-old child is admitted to the hospital for a course of I.V. antibiotics. What should a nurse do before inserting the peripheral I.V. catheter?

Select all that apply.

- ☐ **1.** Explain the procedure to the child immediately before the procedure.
- ☐ **2.** Apply a topical anesthetic to the I.V. site before the procedure.
- ☐ **3.** Ask the child which hand he uses for drawing.
- ☐ **4.** Explain the procedure to the child using abstract terms.
- ☐ **5.** Don't let the child see the equipment to be used in the procedure.
- ☐ **6.** Tell the child that the procedure won't hurt.

Answer: 2, 3

Rationale: Topical anesthetics reduce the pain of a venipuncture. The cream should be applied about 1 hour before the procedure and requires a physician's order. Asking which hand the child draws with helps to identify the dominant hand. The I.V. should be inserted into the opposite extremity so that the child can continue to play and to do homework with minimum disruption. The child should have the procedure explained to him well before it takes place so that he has time to ask questions. Younger school-age children don't have the capability for abstract thinking. The procedure should be explained using simple words and unfamiliar terms should be defined. The child should be shown the equipment that will be used to help ease his anxiety. Although the topical anesthetic will relieve some pain, there's usually some pain or discomfort involved in venipuncture, so the child shouldn't be told otherwise.

Nursing process step: Implementation

Client needs category: Health promotion and maintenance

Client needs subcategory: None

Cognitive level: Application

2. A mother brings her child to the pediatrician's office for evaluation of chronic stomach pain. The mother states that the pain seems to go away when she tells the child that he can stay home from school. The physician diagnoses school phobia. Which other behaviors or symptoms may the child exhibit:

- ☐ **1.** Nausea
- ☐ **2.** Headaches
- ☐ **3.** Weight loss
- ☐ **4.** Dizziness
- ☐ **5.** Fever

Answer: 1, 2, 4

Rationale: Children with school phobia commonly complain of vague symptoms, such as stomachaches, nausea, headaches, and dizziness, to avoid going to school. These symptoms typically don't occur on weekends. A careful history must be taken to identify a pattern of school avoidance. Weight loss and fever are more likely to have a physiological cause and are uncommon in the child with school phobia.

Nursing process step: Analysis

Client needs category: Psychosocial integrity

Client needs subcategory: None

Cognitive level: Analysis

3. A child with sickle cell anemia is being discharged after treatment for a crisis. Which instructions for avoiding future crises should ta nurse provide to the child and his family?

Select all that apply.

- ☐ **1.** Avoid foods high in folic acid.
- ☐ **2.** Drink plenty of fluids.
- ☐ **3.** Use cold packs to relieve joint pain.
- ☐ **4.** Report a sore throat to an adult immediately.
- ☐ **5.** Restrict activity to quiet board games.
- ☐ **6.** Wash hands before meals and after playing.

Answer: 2, 4, 6

Rationale: Fluids should be encouraged to prevent stasis in the bloodstream, which can lead to sickling. Sore throats and all other cold symptoms should be reported promptly because they may indicate the presence of an infection, which can precipitate a crisis (red blood cells sickle and obstruct blood flow to tissues). Children with sickle cell anemia should learn appropriate measures to prevent infection, such as proper hand-washing techniques and good nutrition. Folic acid intake should be encouraged to help support new cell growth; new cells replace fragile sickled cells. Warm packs should be applied to provide comfort and relieve pain; cold packs cause vasoconstriction. The child should maintain an active, normal life but should avoid excessive exercise, which can precipitate an attack. When the child experiences a crisis, he'll typically limit his own activity according to his pain level.

Nursing process step: Planning

Client needs category: Physiological integrity

Client needs subcategory: Reduction of risk potential

Cognitive level: Application

---

4. A nurse is preparing to administer I.V. methylprednisolone sodium succinate (Solu-Medrol) to a child who weighs 42 lb. The order is for 0.03 mg/kg I.V. daily. How many milligrams should the nurse prepare?

_____

Answer: 0.6

Rationale: To perform this dosage calculation, the nurse should first convert the child's weight to kilograms:

$$44 \text{ lb} \div 2.2 \text{ kg/lb} = 20 \text{ kg}.$$

Then she should use this formula to determine the dose:

$$20 \text{ kg} \times 0.03 \text{ mg/kg} = X \text{ mg}$$

$$X = 0.6 \text{ mg}.$$

Nursing process step: Implementation

Client needs category: Physiological integrity

Client needs subcategory: Pharmacological and parenteral therapies

Cognitive level: Application

5. An 8-year-old child has just returned from the operating room after having a tonsillectomy. A nurse is preparing to do a postoperative assessment. The nurse should be alert for which signs and symptoms of bleeding?

Select all that apply.

☐ **1.** Frequent clearing of the throat

☐ **2.** Breathing through the mouth

☐ **3.** Frequent swallowing

☐ **4.** Sleeping for long intervals

☐ **5.** Pulse rate of 98 beats/minute

☐ **6.** Blood-red vomitus

Answer: 1, 3, 6

Rationale: A classic sign of bleeding after tonsillectomy is frequent swallowing; this occurs because blood drips down the back of the throat, tickling it. Other signs include frequent clearing of the throat and vomiting of bright red blood. Vomiting of dark blood may occur if the child swallowed blood during surgery but doesn't indicate postoperative bleeding. Breathing through the mouth is common because of dried secretions in the nares. Sleeping for long intervals is normal after receiving sedation and anesthesia. A pulse rate of 98 beats/minute is in the normal range for this age-group.

Nursing process step: Assessment

Client needs category: Physiological integrity

Client needs subcategory: Reduction of risk potential

Cognitive level: Application

---

6. A 6-year-old child with complaints of fever, malaise, and anorexia is diagnosed with varicella (chickenpox). A nurse teaches the mother how the skin lesions will develop. Place the following descriptions in the order that they will occur as the disease progresses.

| **1.** As initial lesions are crusting over, new lesions form on the trunk and extremities. |
| **2.** Papules develop into clear vesicles on an erythematous base. |
| **3.** Itchy red macules on the face, scalp, and trunk progress to papules. |
| **4.** Vesicles become cloudy and break easily. |
| **5.** Scabs form. |
| |
| |
| |
| |
| |

Answer:

| **3.** Itchy red macules on the face, scalp, and trunk progress to papules. |
| **2.** Papules develop into clear vesicles on an erythematous base. |
| **4.** Vesicles become cloudy and break easily. |
| **5.** Scabs form. |
| **1.** As initial lesions are crusting over, new lesions form on the trunk and extremities. |

Rationale: Fever, malaise, and anorexia occur 24 to 48 hours before a rash develops. The rash begins as itchy red macules on the face, scalp, and trunk. These macules progress to papules, which develop into clear vesicles on an erythematous base. These vesicles become cloudy and break, forming scabs. New lesions continue to form on the trunk and extremities.

Nursing process step: Planning

Client needs category: Physiological integrity

Client needs subcategory: Basic care and comfort

Cognitive level: Analysis

---

7. A nurse is teaching bicycle safety to a child and his parents. Indicate the part of the body on the illustration below that the nurse should tell the clients is most important to protect during bicycle riding.

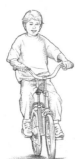

Answer:

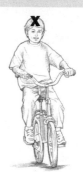

Rationale: A well-fitting helmet that protects the head is the most important safety feature to stress to children and parents. According to the American Academy of Pediatrics, wearing a helmet correctly can prevent or lessen the severity of brain injuries resulting from bicycle crashes.

Nursing process step: Implementation

Client needs category: Physiological integrity

Client needs subcategory: Reduction of risk potential

Cognitive level: Application

---

8. A 10-year-old child visits the pediatrician's office for his annual physical examination. When a nurse asks how he's doing, he becomes quiet and states that his grandmother died last week. Which statements by the child show that he understands the concept of death?

Select all that apply.

☐ **1.** "Death is irreversible and final."

☐ **2.** "All people must die."

☐ **3.** "My grandmother's death has been hard to understand."

☐ **4.** "My grandmother died because she was sick and nothing could make her better."

☐ **5.** "My grandmother is dead, but she'll come back."

☐ **6.** "My grandmother died because someone in the family did something bad."

Answer: 1, 3, 4

Rationale: By age 10, most children know that death is irreversible and final. However, a child may still have difficulty understanding the death of a specific loved one or understanding that children can die. School-age children should be able to identify cause-and-effect relationships, such as when a terminal illness causes someone to die. Adolescents, not school-age children, understand that death is a universal process. Preschoolers see death as temporary and may think of death as a punishment.

Nursing process step: Planning

Client needs category: Health promotion and maintenance

Client needs subcategory: None

Cognitive level: Analysis

9. A child with sickle cell anemia is being treated for a crisis. The physician orders morphine sulfate (Duramorph) 2 mg I.V. The concentration of the vial is 10 mg/1 ml of solution. How many milliliters of solution should the nurse administer?

_____

Rationale: The nurse should calculate the volume to be given using this equation:

$$2 \text{ mg}/X \text{ ml} = 10 \text{ mg}/1 \text{ ml}$$

$$10X = 2$$

$$X = 0.2 \text{ ml}.$$

Nursing process step: Implementation

Client needs category: Physiological integrity

Client needs subcategory: Pharmacological and parenteral therapies

Cognitive level: Application

The adolescent

1. A nurse is caring for an adolescent girl who was admitted to the hospital's medical unit after attempting suicide by ingesting acetaminophen (Tylenol). The nurse should incorporate which interventions into the care plan for this client?

Select all that apply.

☐ **1.** Limit care until the client initiates a conversation.

☐ **2.** Ask the client's parents if they keep firearms in their home.

☐ **3.** Ask the client if she's currently having suicidal thoughts.

☐ **4.** Assist the client with bathing and grooming as needed.

☐ **5.** Inspect the client's mouth after giving oral medications.

☐ **6.** Assure the client that anything she says will be held in strict confidence.

Answer: 2, 3, 4, 5

Rationale: Safety is the primary consideration when caring for suicidal clients. Because firearms are the most common method used in suicides, the client's parents should be taught to lock firearms and ammunition in separate locations and not give the client access to the keys. Safety also includes assessing for current suicidal ideation. Many suicidal people are depressed and don't have the energy to care for themselves, so the client may need assistance with bathing and grooming. Because depressed and suicidal clients may hide pills in their cheeks, the nurse should inspect the client's mouth after giving oral medications. Rather than limit care, the nurse should try to establish a trusting relationship through nursing interventions and therapeutic communication. The client can't be guaranteed confidentiality when self-destructive behavior is an issue.

Nursing process step: Planning

Client needs category: Psychosocial integrity

Client needs subcategory: None

Cognitive level: Application

2. A nurse is teaching an adolescent with inflammatory bowel disease about treatment with corticosteroids. Which adverse effects are concerns for this client?

Select all that apply.

☐ **1.** Acne

☐ **2.** Hirsutism

☐ **3.** Mood swings

☐ **4.** Osteoporosis

☐ **5.** Growth spurts

☐ **6.** Adrenal suppression

Rationale: Adverse effects of corticosteroids include acne, hirsutism, mood swings, osteoporosis, and adrenal suppression. Steroid use in children and adolescents may cause delayed growth, not growth spurts.

Nursing process step: Implementation

Client needs category: Physiological integrity

Client needs subcategory: Pharmacological and parenteral therapies

Cognitive level: Application

---

3. A nurse is caring for a 17-year-old female client with cystic fibrosis who has been admitted to the hospital to receive I.V. antibiotic and respiratory treatment for exacerbation of a lung infection. The client has a number of questions about her future and the consequences of the disease. Which statements about the course of cystic fibrosis are true?

Select all that apply.

☐ **1.** Breast development is commonly delayed.

☐ **2.** The client is at risk for developing diabetes.

☐ **3.** Pregnancy and childbearing aren't affected.

☐ **4.** Normal sexual relationships can be expected.

☐ **5.** Only males carry the gene for the disease.

☐ **6.** By age 20, the client should be able to decrease the frequency of respiratory treatment.

Rationale: Cystic fibrosis delays growth and the onset of puberty. Children with cystic fibrosis tend to be smaller than average size and develop secondary sex characteristics later in life. In addition, they're at risk for developing diabetes mellitus because the pancreatic duct becomes obstructed as pancreatic tissues are destroyed. Clients with cystic fibrosis can expect to have normal sexual relationships, but thick secretions that obstruct the cervix and block sperm entry may impair fertility. Males and females carry the gene for cystic fibrosis. Pulmonary disease commonly progresses as the client ages, requiring additional respiratory treatment, not less.

Nursing process step: Analysis

Client needs category: Physiological integrity

Client needs subcategory: Physiological adaptation

Cognitive level: Analysis

4. A nurse is preparing to administer the first dose of tobramycin (Nebcin) to an adolescent with cystic fibrosis. The order is for 3 mg/kg I.V. daily in three divided doses. The client weighs 99 lb. How many milligrams should the nurse administer per dose?

_____

Answer: 45

Rationale: To perform this dosage calculation, the nurse should first convert the client's weight to kilograms using this formula:

$$1 \text{ kg}/2.2 \text{ lb} = X \text{ kg}/99 \text{ lb}$$

$$2.2X = 99$$

$$X = 45 \text{ kg}.$$

Then she should calculate the client's daily dose using this formula:

$$45 \text{ kg} \times 3 \text{ mg/kg} = 135 \text{ mg}.$$

Finally, the nurse should calculate the divided dose:

$$135 \text{ mg} \div 3 \text{ doses} = 45 \text{ mg/dose}.$$

Nursing process step: Implementation

Client needs category: Physiological integrity

Client needs subcategory: Pharmacological and parenteral therapies

Cognitive level: Application

118   PEDIATRIC NURSING

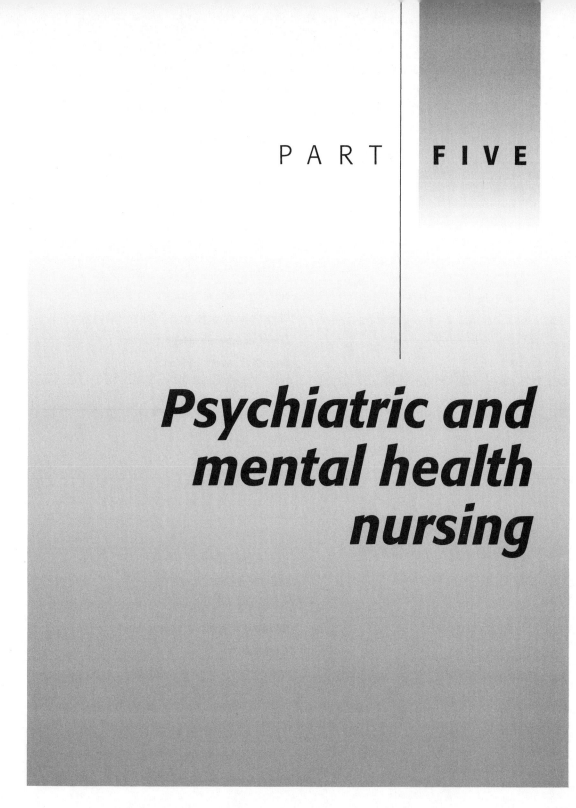

PART FIVE

Psychiatric and mental health nursing

Foundations of psychiatric nursing

1. A client becomes angry and belligerent toward a nurse after speaking on the phone with his mother. The nurse learns that the mother can't visit as expected. Which interventions might the nurse use to help the client deal with his displaced anger?

Select all that apply.

☐ **1.** Explore the client's unmet needs.

☐ **2.** Avoid the client until he apologizes.

☐ **3.** Suggest that the client direct his anger at his mother.

☐ **4.** Invite the client to a quiet place to talk.

☐ **5.** Assist the client in identifying alternate ways of approaching the problem.

> *Answer: 1, 4, 5*

Rationale: Feelings of displacement or directing his anger toward the nurse need to be identified and understood by the client before the caregiver can help guide the client to choose appropriate actions. Avoiding the client or having him direct anger at another person is inappropriate. Approaching the client in a calm manner and offering to assist in the problem-solving process allows the client to identify his needs that are not being met and explore constructive ways of dealing with his anger.

Nursing process step: Implementation

Client needs category: Psychosocial integrity

Client needs subcategory: None

Cognitive level: Application

2. Electroconvulsive therapy (ECT) is an effective treatment for severe depression when which of the following conditions are present?

Select all that apply.

☐ **1.** The client also has dementia.

☐ **2.** The client can't tolerate tricyclic antidepressants.

☐ **3.** The client lives in a long-term care facility.

☐ **4.** The client is undergoing a stressful life change.

☐ **5.** The client is having acute suicidal thoughts.

> *Answer: 2, 5*

Rationale: ECT is used to treat acute depressive illnesses in an attempt to rapidly reverse a life-threatening situation, such as disturbing delusions, agitation, or attempted suicide. If the client can't tolerate tricyclic antidepressants, other medication regimens for depression can take weeks to become effective. ECT usually isn't indicated for situational depression or for clients with dementia. The decision to use ECT isn't based on where the client lives.

Nursing process step: Planning

Client needs category: Psychosocial integrity

Client needs subcategory: None

Cognitive level: Application

3. A nurse knows that her initial approach to a rape victim should aim to decrease the client's anxiety. Which of the following interventions would be appropriate?

Select all that apply.

☐ **1.** Admit the client to the treatment area right away.

☐ **2.** Encourage the client to undergo an examination immediately in order to get it behind her.

☐ **3.** Assure the client that she's safe in the examination room.

☐ **4.** Touch the client early on so that she knows the nurse is supportive.

☐ **5.** Allow a third party to be present if the client requests it.

☐ **6.** Ask "what" questions to determine the type of assault.

Rationale: Immediately admitting a rape victim to the treatment area may help her feel cared for and safe. Allowing a third party to remain with her, if requested, increases her feeling of safety. "What" questions help to clarify what happened in a nonjudgmental way. At a time of great distress, the nurse should pace the interview and examination according to the client's level of comfort. Touching a client who has recently been assaulted may increase her anxiety. The nurse should wait for the client to initiate contact.

Nursing process step: Implementation

Client needs category: Psychosocial integrity

Client needs subcategory: None

Cognitive level: Application

---

4. A nurse is engaging in a therapeutic relationship with a client. Which of the following describe this?

Select all that apply.

☐ **1.** Identify and meet the needs of the client and nurse.

☐ **2.** Help the client explore different problem-solving techniques.

☐ **3.** Encourage the practice of new coping skills.

☐ **4.** Give advice to the client.

☐ **5.** Exchange personal information with the client.

☐ **6.** Discuss the client's feelings with her family members.

Rationale: The goal of a therapeutic relationship is to enhance the personal growth of the client. This is achieved by helping clients explore problem-solving techniques and develop coping skills. Giving advice, exchanging personal information, and striving to meet personal needs of both the nurse and the client are characteristic of social relationships. Discussing the client's feelings with family members is a breach of confidentiality, unless previously approved by the client.

Nursing process step: Implementation

Client needs category: Psychosocial integrity

Client needs subcategory: None

Cognitive level: Analysis

5. A nurse is explaining the Bill of Rights for psychiatric patients to a client who has voluntarily sought admission to an inpatient psychiatric facility. Which of the following rights should the nurse include in the discussion?

Select all that apply.

☐ **1.** Right to select health care team members

☐ **2.** Right to refuse treatment

☐ **3.** Right to a written treatment plan

☐ **4.** Right to obtain disability benefits

☐ **5.** Right to confidentiality

☐ **6.** Right to personal mail

Answer: 2, 3, 5, 6

Rationale: An inpatient client usually receives a copy of the Bill of Rights for psychiatric patients, which includes the right to refuse treatment, have a written treatment plan, have all her medical information kept confidential, and receive mail. However, a client in an inpatient setting cannot select health care team members. A client may apply for disability benefits as a result of a chronic, incapacitating illness; however, disability compensation is not a patient right, and members of a psychiatric institution don't decide who should receive it.

Nursing process step: Implementation

Client needs category: Psychosocial integrity

Client needs subcategory: None

Cognitive level: Application

---

6. In the emergency department, a client reveals to the nurse a lethal plan for committing suicide and agrees to a voluntary admission to the psychiatric unit. Which information should the nurse discuss with the client to answer the question "How long do I have to stay here?"

Select all that apply.

☐ **1.** "You may leave the hospital at any time unless you are suicidal or homicidal or unable to meet your basic needs."

☐ **2.** "Let's talk more after the health care team has assessed you."

☐ **3.** "Once you've signed the papers, you have no say."

☐ **4.** "Because you could hurt yourself, you must be safe before being discharged."

☐ **5.** "You need a lawyer to help you make that decision."

☐ **6.** "There must be a court hearing before you can leave the hospital."

Answer: 1, 2, 4

Rationale: A person who is admitted to a psychiatric hospital voluntarily may sign out of the hospital unless the health care team determines that the person is harmful to himself or others. The health care team evaluates the client's condition before discharge. If there is reason to believe that the client may be harmful to himself or others, a hearing can be held to determine if the admission status should be changed from voluntary to involuntary. The client still has rights after committing himself to a psychiatric unit. The client doesn't need a lawyer to leave the hospital. A court hearing is held only if the client may pose a threat to himself or others and requires further treatment.

Nursing process step: Implementation

Client needs category: Psychosocial integrity

Client needs subcategory: None

Cognitive level: Application

7. A nurse has developed a relationship with a client who has an addiction problem. Which actions would indicate that the therapeutic interaction is in the working phase?

Select all that apply.

☐ **1.** The client discusses how the addiction has contributed to family distress.

☐ **2.** The client reluctantly shares the family history of addiction.

☐ **3.** The client verbalizes difficulty identifying personal strengths.

☐ **4.** The client discusses the financial problems related to the addiction.

☐ **5.** The client expresses uncertainty about meeting with the nurse.

☐ **6.** The client acknowledges the addiction's effects on his children.

Answer: 1, 3, 4, 6

Rationale: Acknowledging the addiction's effects on the family and discussing its financial impact will help the client to identify personal strengths in dealing with addiction and strengthen the therapeutic relationship in the process. Discussing the family history of addiction and expressing uncertainty about meeting the nurse typically happen during the introductory phase of a nurse-client relationship.

Nursing process step: Evaluation

Client needs category: Psychosocial integrity

Client needs subcategory: None

Cognitive level: Application

Anxiety disorders

1. A nurse is caring for a client with agoraphobia. Which of the following signs and symptoms would the nurse expect to find in this client?

Select all that apply.

☐ **1.** Hallucinations

☐ **2.** Panic attacks

☐ **3.** Inability to leave home

☐ **4.** Eating disorders

☐ **5.** Alcohol consumption

☐ **6.** Tobacco use

Answer: 2, 3

Rationale: Agoraphobia is characterized by extreme anxiety and a fear of being in open places. Panic attacks and an inability to leave home are symptoms associated with the disorder. No correlation exists between fear of open spaces and hallucinations, eating disorders, alcohol consumption, or tobacco use.

Nursing process step: Assessment

Client needs category: Psychosocial integrity

Client needs subcategory: None

Cognitive level: Analysis

2. A client is being seen in the clinic after returning from military service abroad. The nurse is aware that posttraumatic stress disorder (PTSD) can be acute or chronic. Which of the following statements about PTSD are accurate?

Select all that apply.

☐ **1.** PTSD is a syndrome that affects only those who have experienced traumatic episodes during war.

☐ **2.** PTSD is characterized by nightmares and flashbacks.

☐ **3.** Hypervigilance is characteristic of clients with PTSD.

☐ **4.** Substance abuse is a common coping mechanism used by clients with PTSD.

☐ **5.** Psychotic episodes can occur in clients with PTSD.

☐ **6.** Clients with PTSD may complain of feeling empty inside.

Answer: 2, 3, 4, 5, 6

Rationale: Although PTSD is commonly associated with combat, it can manifest itself after any kind of trauma. If symptoms occur within 6 months of the traumatic event, the disorder is considered acute. If symptoms occur more than 6 months after the traumatic event, PTSD is considered delayed or chronic. PTSD is characterized by nightmares or flashbacks. Clients are hypervigilant but typically describe themselves as "empty inside." Sometimes, the events can present as a psychotic episode. Substance abuse is a common "symptom" used for coping.

Nursing process step: Assessment

Client needs category: Psychosocial integrity

Client needs subcategory: None

Cognitive level: Analysis

---

3. An 8-year-old child diagnosed with obsessive-compulsive disorder is admitted to a psychiatric facility. Which of the following behaviors would a nurse assessing the client characterize as compulsions?

Select all that apply.

☐ **1.** Checking and rechecking that the television is turned off before going to school

☐ **2.** Repeatedly washing the hands

☐ **3.** Brushing teeth three times per day

☐ **4.** Routinely climbing up and down a flight of stairs three times before leaving the house

☐ **5.** Feeding the dog the same meal every day

☐ **6.** Wanting to play the same video game each night

Answer: 1, 2, 4

Rationale: Compulsions involve symbolic rituals that relieve anxiety when they are performed. The disorder is caused by anxiety from obsessive thoughts and acts are seen as irrational. Examples are repeatedly checking the television set, washing hands, or climbing stairs. An activity, such as playing the same video game each night, may be indicative of normal development for a school-age child. Frequent teethbrushing and feeding the dog a consistent meal daily are not abnormal.

Nursing process step: Assessment

Client needs category: Psychosocial integrity

Client needs subcategory: None

Cognitive level: Analysis

4. A client with the nursing diagnosis of *Fear related to being embarrassed in the presence of others* exhibits symptoms of social phobia. What nursing outcomes should the nurse establish for this client?

Select all that apply.

☐ **1.** Manage her fear in group situations.

☐ **2.** Develop a plan to avoid situations that may cause stress.

☐ **3.** Verbalize feelings that occur in stressful situations.

☐ **4.** Develop a plan for responding to stressful situations.

☐ **5.** Deny feelings that may contribute to irrational fears.

☐ **6.** Use suppression to deal with underlying fears.

Answer: 1, 3, 4

Rationale: Improving stress management skills, verbalizing feelings, and anticipating and planning for stressful situations are adaptive responses to stress. Avoidance, denial, and suppression are maladaptive defense mechanisms.

Nursing process step: Planning

Client needs category: Psychosocial integrity

Client needs subcategory: None

Cognitive level: Application

---

5. A nurse recognizes improvement in a client with the nursing diagnosis of *Ineffective role performance related to the need to perform rituals*. Which of the following behaviors indicates improvement?

Select all that apply.

☐ **1.** The client refrains from performing rituals during stress.

☐ **2.** The client says that he uses "thought stopping" when obsessive thoughts occur.

☐ **3.** The client verbalizes the relationship between stress and ritualistic behaviors.

☐ **4.** The client avoids stressful situations.

☐ **5.** The client rationalizes ritualistic behavior.

☐ **6.** The client performs ritualistic behaviors in private.

Answer: 1, 2, 3

Rationale: Refraining from performing rituals demonstrates that the client manages stress appropriately. Using "thought stopping" demonstrates the client's ability to employ appropriate interventions for obsessive thoughts. Verbalizing the relationship between stress and behaviors indicates that the client understands the disease process. Avoiding stressful situations and rationalizing or hiding ritualistic behaviors are maladaptive methods of managing stress and anxiety.

Nursing process step: Evaluation

Client needs category: Psychosocial integrity

Client needs subcategory: None

Cognitive level: Analysis

6. A recent diagnosis of cancer has caused a client severe anxiety. Which of the following interventions should the nurse include in the care plan?

Select all that apply.

☐ **1.** Maintain a calm, nonthreatening environment.

☐ **2.** Explain relevant aspects of chemotherapy.

☐ **3.** Encourage the client to verbalize her concerns regarding the diagnosis.

☐ **4.** Encourage the client to use deep-breathing exercises and other relaxation techniques during periods of increased stress.

☐ **5.** Provide distractions for the client during periods of stress.

☐ **6.** Teach the stages of grieving to the client.

Answer: 1, 3, 4

Rationale: During periods of acute stress, interventions that help the client regain control will help the client master this new threat. Providing a calm, nonthreatening environment and encouraging verbalization of concerns will help the client face the unknown. Relaxation techniques have a physiologic and psychological effect in calming the client, which in turn allows further exploration of thoughts and feelings as well as problem solving. The ability to learn is limited during extreme stress, so teaching wouldn't be effective at this stage. Providing distractions would be ineffective at this point in the grief process.

Nursing process step: Implementation

Client needs category: Psychosocial integrity

Client needs subcategory: None

Cognitive level: Application

Mood, adjustment, and dementia disorders

1. A nurse is conducting a group session for children and adolescents who have been diagnosed with depression. Which of the following behaviors would a nurse expect to see in this group?

Select all that apply.

☐ **1.** Delusions

☐ **2.** Anxiety

☐ **3.** Sadness

☐ **4.** Irritability

☐ **5.** Somatic symptoms, such as headache or stomachache

☐ **6.** Suicidal thoughts

Answer: 2, 4, 5, 6

Rationale: Children and adolescents with depression commonly experience anxiety and irritability (rather than sadness) as well as somatic symptoms. Suicide is a serious risk in these age-groups. These age-groups seldom experience psychotic symptoms. If psychotic symptoms do occur, they are more likely to be auditory hallucinations than delusions.

Nursing process step: Assessment

Client needs category: Psychosocial integrity

Client needs subcategory: None

Cognitive level: Analysis

2. A client is diagnosed with dysthymia. A nurse is aware that which of the following symptoms and characteristics are associated with dysthymia?

Select all that apply.

☐ **1.** Insomnia or hypersomnia

☐ **2.** Delusions or hallucinations

☐ **3.** Suicidal thoughts

☐ **4.** Onset of symptoms within a 2-week period

☐ **5.** Symptoms that occur in the winter and resolve in spring

☐ **6.** Appetite disturbance

Answer: 1, 3, 6

Rationale: Sleep and appetite disturbances and suicidal thoughts can appear in clients with dysthymia or major depressive disorders. Onset of symptoms are gradual and may appear over weeks or months. Delusions and other psychotic symptoms may occur in major depression, but don't occur in dysthymia, a milder and more chronic mood disorder. Episodes of depression occurring solely in winter are indicative of seasonal affective disorder.

Nursing process step: Assessment

Client needs category: Psychosocial integrity

Client needs subcategory: None

Cognitive level: Analysis

---

3. A nurse is developing a care plan for a client with acute mania. Place the following behaviors in the order in which they occur as the client develops acute mania.

| **1.** Delusions of grandeur |
| **2.** Relevant, calm speech patterns |
| **3.** Highly productive and competitive in work and leisure activities |
| **4.** Easily irritated |
| **5.** Poor judgement and impulse control |

| |
| |
| |
| |
| |

Answer:

| **2.** Relevant, calm speech patterns |
| **3.** Highly productive and competitive in work and leisure activities |
| **4.** Easily irritated |
| **1.** Delusions of grandeur |
| **5.** Poor judgement and impulse control |

Rationale: Relevant and calm speech patterns are indicative of normal behavior. Once mania begins, the client may become highly productive and competitive in all activities. Sleep is not a priority. As mania progresses, emotional manifestations heighten and the client is easily irritated, begins to have delusions of grandeur, and may require medication (chemical restraint) to reduce restlessness and agitation. Client safety is the primary goal due to poor judgement and impulse control.

Nursing process step: Assessment

Client needs category: Psychosocial integrity

Client needs subcategory: None

Cognitive level: Analysis

4. A physician prescribes lithium for a client diagnosed with bipolar disorder. Which of the following topics should a nurse cover when teaching the client?

Select all that apply.

☐ **1.** Potential for addiction

☐ **2.** Signs and symptoms of drug toxicity

☐ **3.** Potential for tardive dyskinesia

☐ **4.** Importance of a low-tyramine diet

☐ **5.** Need to consistently monitor blood levels

☐ **6.** Amount of time that may be needed for mood changes to occur

Answer: 2, 5, 6

Rationale: Client education should cover the signs and symptoms of drug toxicity, the need to report them to the physician, and the need for regular monitoring of drug blood levels. The nurse should also inform the client that mood changes may not be apparent for 7 to 21 days after treatment is initiated. Lithium doesn't have addictive properties and doesn't cause tardive dyskinesia. Tyramine is a potential concern to clients who are also taking monoamine-oxidase inhibitors.

Nursing process step: Implementation

Client needs category: Physiological integrity

Client needs subcategory: Pharmacological and parenteral therapies

Cognitive level: Application

5. After interviewing a client diagnosed with recurrent depression, a nurse determines the client's potential to commit suicide. Which factors listed below might contribute to the client's potential for suicide?

Select all that apply.

☐ **1.** Psychomotor retardation

☐ **2.** Impulsive behaviors

☐ **3.** Overwhelming feelings of guilt

☐ **4.** Chronic, debilitating illness

☐ **5.** Decreased physical activity

☐ **6.** Repression of anger

Answer: 2, 3, 4, 6

Rationale: Impulsive behavior, overwhelming guilt, chronic illness, and anger repression are factors that contribute to suicide potential. Psychomotor retardation and decreased activity are symptoms of depression but don't typically lead to suicide because the client doesn't have the energy to harm himself.

Nursing process step: Analysis

Client needs category: Psychosocial integrity

Client needs subcategory: None

Cognitive level: Analysis

6. A nurse is assessing a client who talks freely about feeling depressed. During the interaction, the nurse hears the client state, "Things will never change." What other indications of hopelessness would the nurse look for?

Select all that apply.

☐ **1.** Bouts of anger

☐ **2.** Periods of irritability

☐ **3.** Preoccupation with delusions

☐ **4.** Feelings of worthlessness

☐ **5.** Self-destructive behaviors

☐ **6.** Auditory hallucinations

Answer: 1, 2, 4, 5

Rationale: Clients who are depressed and feeling hopeless are often irritable and express inappropriate anger, feelings of worthlessness, and suicidal thoughts. In addition, they may demonstrate self-destructive behaviors. Preoccupation with delusions and auditory hallucinations is generally seen in clients with schizophrenia or other psychotic disorders rather than in those expressing hopelessness.

Nursing process step: Assessment

Client needs category: Psychosocial integrity

Client needs subcategory: None

Cognitive level: Analysis

---

7. A nurse interviews the family of a client hospitalized with severe depression and suicidal ideation. What family assessment information is essential in formulating an effective plan of care?

Select all that apply.

☐ **1.** Physical pain

☐ **2.** Personal responsibilities

☐ **3.** Employment skills

☐ **4.** Communication patterns

☐ **5.** Role expectations

☐ **6.** Current family stressors

Answer: 4, 5, 6

Rationale: When working with the family of a depressed client, it's helpful for the nurse to be aware of the family's communication style, role expectations, and current family stressors. This information can help to identify family difficulties and teaching points that could benefit the client and the family. Information concerning physical pain, personal responsibilities, and employment skills wouldn't be helpful because these areas aren't directly related to their experience of having a depressed family member.

Nursing process step: Planning

Client needs category: Psychosocial integrity

Client needs subcategory: None

Cognitive level: Analysis

8. A client is prescribed sertraline (Zoloft), a selective serotonin reuptake inhibitor. Which adverse effects would the nurse include when creating a medication teaching plan?

Select all that apply.

☐ **1.** Agitation

☐ **2.** Agranulocytosis

☐ **3.** Sleep disturbance

☐ **4.** Intermittent tachycardia

☐ **5.** Dry mouth

☐ **6.** Seizures

Answer: 1, 3, 5

Rationale: Common adverse effects of sertraline are agitation, sleep disturbance, and dry mouth. Agranulocytosis, intermittent tachycardia, and seizures are adverse effects of clozapine (Clozaril).

Nursing process step: Planning

Client needs category: Physiological integrity

Client needs subcategory: Pharmacological and parenteral therapies

Cognitive level: Application

---

9. A nurse is assessing a client for dementia. What history would the nurse expect to find in a client with dementia?

Select all that apply.

☐ **1.** The progression of symptoms is slow.

☐ **2.** The client admits to feelings of sadness.

☐ **3.** The client acts apathetic and pessimistic.

☐ **4.** The family can't determine when the symptoms first appeared.

☐ **5.** The client exhibits basic personality changes.

☐ **6.** The client has great difficulty paying attention to others.

Answer: 1, 4, 5, 6

Rationale: Dementia is characterized by a slow onset of symptoms, which makes it difficult to determine when symptoms first occurred. It progresses to noticeable changes in the individual's personality and impaired ability to pay attention to other people. Sadness, apathy, and pessimism are symptoms of depression.

Nursing process step: Assessment

Client needs category: Health promotion and maintenance

Client needs subcategory: None

Cognitive level: Analysis

10. A client has been diagnosed with an adjustment disorder with mixed anxiety and depression. What are the primary nursing diagnoses the nurse associates with an adjustment disorder?

Select all that apply.

☐ **1.** Activity intolerance

☐ **2.** Impaired social interaction

☐ **3.** Self-esteem disturbance

☐ **4.** Personal identity disturbance

☐ **5.** Acute confusion

☐ **6.** Impaired memory

Answer: 2, 3

Rationale: A client with an adjustment disorder is likely to exhibit impaired social interaction and self-esteem disturbance. Activity intolerance, personal identity disturbance, acute confusion, and impaired memory aren't related to an adjustment disorder.

Nursing process step: Analysis

Client needs category: Psychosocial integrity

Client needs subcategory: None

Cognitive level: Analysis

Psychotic disorders

1. A nurse is assessing a new client and notices clang associations in his speech pattern. This symptom is commonly seen in clients with which of the following disorders?

Select all that apply.

☐ **1.** Multiple personality disorder

☐ **2.** Schizophrenia

☐ **3.** Narcolepsy

☐ **4.** Mania

☐ **5.** Organic disorders

☐ **6.** Intermittent explosive disorder

Answer: 2, 4, 5

Rationale: This speech pattern, characterized by meaningless rhymes, is found most commonly in clients with schizophrenia but may also be present in clients with bipolar disorder (during the manic phase) or organic disorders. It's not characteristic of personality disorders, narcolepsy, or explosive disorders.

Nursing process step: Assessment

Client needs category: Psychosocial integrity

Client needs subcategory: None

Cognitive level: Analysis

2. A nurse is monitoring a client who appears to be hallucinating. The client is gesturing at a figure on the television. He appears agitated and his speech contains paranoid content. Which of the following nursing interventions are appropriate?

Select all that apply.

☐ **1.** In a firm voice, instruct the client to stop the behavior.

☐ **2.** Reassure the client that he's not in any danger.

☐ **3.** Acknowledge the presence of the hallucinations.

☐ **4.** Instruct other team members to ignore the client's behavior.

☐ **5.** Immediately implement physical restraints.

☐ **6.** Give simple commands in a calm voice.

Answer: 2, 3, 6

Rationale: Using a calm voice and giving simple commands, the nurse should reassure the client that he is safe. She shouldn't challenge the client; rather, she should acknowledge his hallucinatory experience. It is not appropriate to request that the client stop the behavior. Ignoring behavior will not reduce agitation. Implementing restraints is not warranted at this time. Although the client is agitated, he doesn't appear to be at risk for harming himself or others.

Nursing process step: Implementation

Client needs category: Psychosocial integrity

Client needs subcategory: None

Cognitive level: Application

---

3. A client with schizophrenia is taking the atypical antipsychotic medication clozapine (Clozaril). Which of the following signs and symptoms suggest that the client may be experiencing an adverse effect associated with this medication?

Select all that apply.

☐ **1.** Sore throat

☐ **2.** Pill-rolling movements

☐ **3.** Polyuria

☐ **4.** Fever

☐ **5.** Polydipsia

☐ **6.** Orthostatic hypotension

Answer: 1, 4

Rationale: Sore throat, fever, and the sudden onset of other flulike symptoms are signs of agranulocytosis, an adverse effect of clozapine. The condition is caused by a deficiency of granulocytes (a type of white blood cell), which causes the individual to be susceptible to infection. The client's white blood cell count should be monitored at least weekly during clozapine treatment. Extrapyramidal effects, such as pill-rolling, either do not occur or occur at a much lesser rate with the atypical antipsychotic medications. Polydipsia (excessive thirst) and polyuria (increased urination) are common adverse effects of lithium. Orthostatic hypotension is an adverse effect of tricyclic antidepressants.

Nursing process step: Assessment

Client needs category: Physiological integrity

Client needs subcategory: Pharmacological and parenteral therapies

Cognitive level: Application

---

4. A delusional client says to a nurse, "I am the Easter bunny" and insists that the nurse refer to him as such. The belief appears to be fixed and unchanging. Which of the following nursing interventions should the nurse implement when working with this client?

Select all that apply.

☐ **1.** Consistently use the client's name in interactions.

☐ **2.** Smile at the humor of the situation.

☐ **3.** Agree that the client is the Easter bunny.

☐ **4.** Logically point out why the client could not be the Easter bunny.

☐ **5.** Provide an as-needed medication.

☐ **6.** Provide the client with structured activities.

Answer: 1, 6

Rationale: This client needs continuous reality-based orientation, so the nurse should use the client's name in any interaction. Structured activities can help the client refocus and resolve his delusion. The nurse shouldn't contribute to the delusion by smiling at the comment or agreeing with the client. Logical arguments and an as-needed medication aren't likely to change the client's beliefs.

Nursing process step: Implementation

Client needs category: Psychosocial integrity

Client needs subcategory: None

Cognitive level: Application

---

5. A physician starts a client on the antipsychotic medication haloperidol (Haldol). The nurse is aware that this medication has extrapyramidal adverse effects. Which of the following measures should the nurse take during haloperidol administration?

Select all that apply.

☐ **1.** Review subcutaneous injection technique.

☐ **2.** Closely monitor vital signs, especially temperature.

☐ **3.** Observe for increased pacing and restlessness.

☐ **4.** Monitor blood glucose levels.

☐ **5.** Provide the client with hard candy.

☐ **6.** Monitor for signs and symptoms of urticaria.

Answer: 2, 3, 5

Rationale: Neuroleptic malignant syndrome is a life-threatening extrapyramidal adverse effect of antipsychotic medications such as haloperidol. It's associated with a rapid increase in temperature. The most common extrapyramidal adverse effect, akathisia, is a form of psychomotor restlessness that is often exhibited as pacing. Haloperidol and the anticholinergic medications that are provided to alleviate its extrapyramidal effects can result in dry mouth. Providing the client with hard candy to suck on can help alleviate this problem. Haloperidol isn't given subcutaneously and doesn't affect blood glucose levels. Urticaria is not usually associated with haloperidol administration.

Nursing process step: Planning

Client needs category: Physiological integrity

Client needs subcategory: Pharmacological and parenteral therapies

Cognitive level: Analysis

6. A nurse is planning to teach a psychiatric assistant class about antipsychotic medications. The students should be taught that which of the following symptoms might occur within the first few weeks of treatment with these medications?

Select all that apply.

☐ **1.** Acute dystonic reactions

☐ **2.** Akathisia

☐ **3.** Tardive dyskinesia

☐ **4.** Neuroleptic malignant syndrome

☐ **5.** Hearing loss

☐ **6.** Orthostatic hypotension

Answer: 1, 2, 4, 6

Rationale: Acute dystonia, akathisia, neuroleptic malignant syndrome, and orthostatic hypotension can occur during the first few weeks of treatment with antipsychotic drugs. Tardive dyskinesia doesn't typically occur until at least 6 months after starting treatment. Hearing loss isn't an adverse effect of antipsychotic drugs.

Nursing process step: Assessment

Client needs category: Psychosocial integrity

Client needs subcategory: None

Cognitive level: Analysis

---

7. A nurse is working with a client with schizophrenia who is experiencing auditory hallucinations. Place the following interventions in the order that best prevents exacerbation of the client's anxiety.

| **1.** Ask the client, "What are you experiencing right now?" |
| **2.** Encourage the client to tell you about the history of his hallucinations. |
| **3.** Tell the client "I'd like to spend time with you to discuss your hallucinations. Is that okay with you?" |
| **4.** Ask the client if he has recently taken drugs or alcohol. |

Answer:

| **3.** Tell the client "I'd like to spend time with you to discuss your hallucinations. Is that okay with you?" |
| **1.** Ask the client, "What are you experiencing right now?" |
| **4.** Ask the client if he has recently taken drugs or alcohol. |
| **2.** Encourage the client to tell you about the history of his hallucinations. |

Rationale: Asking the client if he'll discuss the hallucinations promotes trust, an essential first step in communicating with hallucinating clients. When the client relates his hallucinations, the nurse should observe for nonverbal cues, such as the client's eyes looking around the room. Asking the client about these observations will help promote understanding of the symptoms, increase trust, and decrease the client's perception that the nurse can read his mind. Asking the client if he has recently taken drugs or alcohol helps determine the source of the current experience. Once trust is established, the client will be more comfortable discussing the history of his hallucinations, such as when the voices started. This step will be beneficial in helping him manage the present.

Nursing process step: Intervention

Client needs category: Psychosocial integrity

Client needs subcategory: None

Cognitive level: Application

8. A client with schizophrenia asks a nurse to explain the causes of the disorder. Knowing that an overactive dopamine system in the brain is one of the leading causes of schizophrenia, the nurse says that excessive dopamine activity is responsible for which of the following symptoms?

Select all that apply.

☐ **1.** Hallucinations

☐ **2.** Withdrawn behavior

☐ **3.** Grandiosity

☐ **4.** Delusional thinking

☐ **5.** Excessive tearfulness

☐ **6.** Hypotension

Answer: 1, 3, 4

Rationale: Hallucinations, grandiosity, and delusional thinking are attributable to the effects of excessive dopamine activity. Withdrawn behavior isn't associated with dopamine. Excessive tearfulness and hypotension aren't commonly associated with schizophrenia or dopamine activity.

Nursing process step: Assessment

Client needs category: Psychosocial integrity

Client needs subcategory: None

Cognitive level: Analysis

Substance abuse, eating disorders, and impulse control disorders

1. A nurse is assessing a client who has been diagnosed with bulimia nervosa. The nurse is aware that which of the following characteristics accompanies eating binges?

Select all that apply.

☐ **1.** Guilt

☐ **2.** Dental caries

☐ **3.** Self-induced vomiting

☐ **4.** Weight loss

☐ **5.** Normal weight

☐ **6.** Introverted behavior

Answer: 1, 2, 3, 5

Rationale: Guilt, dental caries, self-induced vomiting, and normal weight are associated with bulimia nervosa. Weight loss and introverted behavior are associated with anorexia nervosa.

Nursing process step: Assessment

Client needs category: Psychosocial integrity

Client needs subcategory: None

Cognitive level: Analysis

2. Clients with opioid addiction who are in withdrawal typically present with which of the following signs and symptoms?

Select all that apply.

☐ **1.** Abdominal cramps

☐ **2.** Dry, warm skin

☐ **3.** Rhinorrhea

☐ **4.** Dilated pupils

☐ **5.** Hypersomnia

☐ **6.** Feeling of hunger

Answer: 1, 3, 4

Rationale: Opioid withdrawal commonly manifests as abdominal cramps, rhinorrhea, dilated pupils, and anorexia (not hunger). Insomnia (not hypersomnia), and diaphoresis (not dry, warm skin), are also common.

Nursing process step: Assessment

Client needs category: Physiological integrity

Client needs subcategory: Pharmacological and parenteral therapies

Cognitive level: Analysis

---

3. A nurse is assessing a client who recently arrived in the emergency department. She's concerned that the client may be under the influence of amphetamines. Which of the following symptoms can indicate amphetamine usage?

Select all that apply.

☐ **1.** Depressed affect

☐ **2.** Diaphoresis

☐ **3.** Shallow respirations

☐ **4.** Hypotension

☐ **5.** Tremors

☐ **6.** Dilated pupils

Answer: 2, 3, 5, 6

Rationale: A client under the influence of amphetamines may present with euphoria, diaphoresis, shallow respirations, dilated pupils, dry mouth, anorexia, tachycardia, hypertension, hyperthermia, tremors, seizures, and altered mental status. A depressed affect and hypotension aren't associated with this disorder.

Nursing process step: Assessment

Client needs category: Physiological integrity

Client needs subcategory: Pharmacological and parenteral therapies

Cognitive level: Application

4. The nurse is caring for an anorexic client with a nursing diagnosis of *Imbalanced nutrition: Less than body requirements* related to dysfunctional eating patterns. Which of the following interventions would be supportive for this client?

Select all that apply.

☐ **1.** Provide small, frequent meals.

☐ **2.** Monitor weight gain.

☐ **3.** Allow the client to skip meals until the antidepressant levels are therapeutic.

☐ **4.** Encourage the client to keep a journal.

☐ **5.** Monitor the client during meals and for 1 hour afterward.

☐ **6.** Encourage the client to eat three substantial meals per day.

Answer: 1, 2, 4, 5

Rationale: Because they're engaged in self-starvation, clients with anorexia rarely can tolerate large meals three times per day. Small, frequent meals may be tolerated better and they provide a way to gradually increase daily caloric intake. The nurse should monitor the client's weight carefully because a client with anorexia may try to hide weight loss. The client may be afraid to express her feelings; keeping a journal can serve as an outlet for these feelings, which can assist recovery. A client with anorexia is already underweight and shouldn't be permitted to skip meals.

Nursing process step: Implementation

Client needs category: Psychosocial integrity

Client needs subcategory: None

Cognitive level: Analysis

---

5. When assessing a client diagnosed with impulse control disorder, the nurse observes violent, aggressive, and assaultive behavior. Which of the following assessment data is the nurse also likely to find?

Select all that apply.

☐ **1.** The client functions well in other areas of his life.

☐ **2.** The degree of aggressiveness is out of proportion to the stressor.

☐ **3.** The violent behavior is usually justified by a stressor.

☐ **4.** The client has a history of parental alcoholism and a chaotic, abusive family life.

☐ **5.** The client has no remorse about the inability to control his behavior.

Answer: 1, 2, 4

Rationale: A client with an impulse control disorder who displays violent, aggressive, and assaultive behavior generally functions well in other areas of his life. The degree of aggressiveness is out of proportion to the stressor, and he frequently has a history of parental alcoholism and a chaotic family life. The client often verbalizes sincere remorse and guilt for the aggressive behavior.

Nursing process step: Assessment

Client needs category: Psychosocial integrity

Client needs subcategory: None

Cognitive level: Application

6. A nurse is caring for a client who has borderline personality disorder. Which of the following interventions are appropriate for clients with this disorder?

Select all that apply.

☐ **1.** Providing antianxiety medications

☐ **2.** Providing emotional consistency

☐ **3.** Exploring anger in appropriate ways

☐ **4.** Encouraging independence as soon as possible

☐ **5.** Promoting gradual separation and individuation

☐ **6.** Ensuring the client's safety

Answer: 2, 3, 5, 6

Rationale: In clients with borderline personalities, the primary goal is to ensure a safe environment. As the client begins to learn how to manage his behavior, suicide still remains a risk. A key intervention includes providing emotional support that is consistent. The client needs to learn how to manage anger effectively and begins to need less support as he separates and develops his individual coping behaviors. Antianxiety drugs are reserved for clinical emergencies.

Nursing process step: Assessment

Client needs category: Psychosocial integrity

Client needs subcategory: None

Cognitive level: Application

7. A client is prescribed chlordiazepoxide (Librium) as needed to control the symptoms of alcohol withdrawal. Which of the following symptoms may indicate the need for an additional dose of this medication?

Select all that apply.

☐ **1.** Tachycardia

☐ **2.** Mood swings

☐ **3.** Elevated blood pressure and temperature

☐ **4.** Piloerection

☐ **5.** Tremors

☐ **6.** Increasing anxiety

Answer: 1, 3, 5, 6

Rationale: Benzodiazepines, such as chlordiazepoxide, are usually administered based on elevations in heart rate, blood pressure, and temperature as well as on the presence of tremors and increasing anxiety. Mood swings are expected during the withdrawal period and are not an indication for further medication administration. Piloerection is not a symptom of alcohol withdrawal.

Nursing process step: Evaluation

Client needs category: Physiological integrity

Client needs subcategory: Pharmacological and parenteral therapies

Cognitive level: Analysis